A Donor Insemination Guide:
Written *By* and *For*
Lesbian Women

Alice Street Editions

Judith P. Stelboum
Editor-in-Chief

Alice Street Editions provides a voice for established as well as up-and-coming lesbian writers, reflecting the diversity of lesbian interests, ethnicities, ages, and class. This cutting-edge series of novels, memoirs, and non-fiction writing welcomes the opportunity to present controversial views, explore multicultural ideas, encourage debate, and inspire creativity from a variety of lesbian perspectives. Through enlightening, illuminating, and provocative writing, Alice Street Editions can make a significant contribution to the visibility and accessibility of lesbian writing, and bring lesbian-focused writing to a wider audience. Recognizing our own desires and ideas in print is life sustaining, acknowledging the reality of who we are, our place in the world, individually and collectively.

Judith P. Stelboum
Editor-in-Chief
Alice Street Editions

A Donor Insemination Guide:
Written *By* and *For*
Lesbian Women

Marie Mohler, MA
Lacy Frazer, PsyD

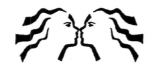

Alice Street Editions

Harrington Park Press
New York • London • Oxford

Published by

Alice Street Editions, Harrington Park Press®, an imprint of The Haworth Press, Inc., 10 Alice Street, Binghamton, NY 13904-1580 USA (www.HaworthPress.com).

Cover design by Thomas J. Mayshock Jr.

Mohler, Marie.
    A donor insemination guide : written by and for lesbian women / Marie Mohler and Lacy Frazer.
      p. cm.
    Includes bibliographical references.
    ISBN 1-56023-226-9 (hard : alk. paper)–ISBN 1-56023-227-7 (pbk. : alk. paper)
    1. Artificial insemination, Human. 2. Lesbian mothers. I. Frazer, Lacy. II. Title.
RG134 .M64 2001
618.1'78–dc21

2001046227

CONTENTS

To our beautiful sons, Jack and Joseph, who have taught us the meaning of unconditional love. Someday you will read this book and know how incredibly happy and proud we are to be your moms.

Foreword

Lesbian women and couples face unique and difficult challenges in fulfilling their desire for children. This comprehensive book explores subtle issues of donor insemination and other aspects of lesbian motherhood that could easily be unanticipated. Marie Mohler and Lacy Frazer have not only researched the utter depths of their topic, but lived it as well. Their journey was made with great fortitude and bravery, and they generously give the wisdom of their experience to you in this book.

That both authors are mental health professionals is very apparent, instilling an emotional and intellectual depth that is immensely helpful. It spans from the very technical aspects of donor insemination and fertility awareness to issues of donor options, love and mutual support, legal questions, and much more. Lacy Frazer's chapter on Parenting Today should be read by all parents.

As you read this book, and refer to it time and again, you will join me in thanking the authors for a wonderful contribution to the knowledge of reproduction, and for their dedication to lesbian motherhood.

Margaret Nofziger
Author and fertility awareness expert

Preface

Many moons ago, it seems, Lacy and I made the decision to actively begin the donor insemination process. The decision to start a family was easy, but the research involved in understanding and negotiating the process was very difficult. We gathered every resource we could find, took chapters of information from different books, and put a plan into motion. Piecemealing our information was a long and tiring process. This fact, combined with the number of setbacks we experienced due to our own inexperience and lack of knowledge, as well as doctor insensitivity and misguidance, led us to write this book. With each month's failure to conceive, we found peace in channeling our frustrations into a plan to provide a resource guide that would prevent other lesbians from having to continuously "reinvent the wheel," and that would also provide validation for this incredible rite of passage.

This book was conceived during the peak of our greatest donor insemination stress and frustration. While this work can serve to validate *any* woman's quest for parenthood through alternative reproduction methods, it was especially written to reach the lesbian reader struggling with the how-to's of becoming pregnant through donor insemination (DI). We welcome both lesbian and heterosexual women into the world of donor insemination to absorb our message as it relates to your needs.

In writing this book, we intend to provide a comprehensive guide through the practical, legal, and emotional issues involved in the donor insemination process. However, there are several limitations to this guide. First and foremost, it is important to state that Lacy and I are not medical doctors, and the information being provided is derived from our search and summation of related literature as well as our own experiences. Thus, please consult a physician should you seek additional information concerning any medical issues, such as infertility, fertility medications, and additional treatments. In addition, it should be stated that we are not attorneys, and we therefore encourage you to explore any and all information regarding the adoption, guardianship, and custody laws *in your state*. The information provided is a result of our own information gathering, contact with attorneys, and personal experiences. If you find that you need further legal guidance, or if something in what we have stated does not ring true for your particular circumstances, we encourage you to meet with an attorney who is versed in the legal nuances of donor insemination and adoption issues.

It is important also to mention that the names of the women whose donor insemination experiences are shared in this book have been altered in order to protect their identities and confidentiality.

Additionally, you will find that we chronicled the donor insemination process through the eyes of women who have had to work extensively with physicians for their inseminations. While there are many women who will perform "at-home" inseminations and parallel the old-fashioned way of getting pregnant, working with a physician has the potential to present additional DI issues that we find necessary to explore in order to prepare those who choose the doctor-assisted insemination path. We recommend your reading all of the material, although we understand that some of the issues presented will not match *every* individual's experience of DI.

And finally, although Lacy and I have an inherent support system in each other as a committed couple, we realize there are single lesbian women who will also choose this path to conception. As with heterosexual parents, similarities *and* differences will likely present themselves for single lesbians as compared to coupled women. The salient differences are often associated with the additional demands on the single parent, given that there is only one person handling all responsibilities. For the single lesbian woman researching DI, these issues include her financial readiness and ability to support the dollar demands of the DI process, her emotional and physical health, energy, and resilience, and her access to open, receptive, and active support systems. In addition, the logistics associated with the scheduling challenges of being the sole provider may add secondary strain to parenting as a single lesbian. Thus, while single lesbian women may find themselves experiencing the very common ups and downs associated with DI and life-long parenting, they may have heightened emotional highs and lows in the absence of an equal partner to share/diffuse the stress and responsibilities. Based on our experience of DI, we suggest that even the most capable, confident, and financially stable woman consider choosing a donor insemination coach or partner with whom she can ride out the daily physical and emotional storms inherent in this process. For committed couples and single lesbian women alike, the partner/coach will need to be communicative, open, and actively involved in the DI experience, including being sensitive to the heightened needs of the "mommy vessel." This directive will be reinforced throughout the book.

We have found great healing and satisfaction in bringing this book to life. The women that we have encountered who have experienced donor insemination and/or fertility issues have reinforced the great need to have a supportive resource in place to validate the *lesbian experience of donor insemination*. Too often we have had to read self-help books or stories about heterosexual couples struggling with conception, and rearrange the material so that its message can apply to our lives. *A Donor Insemination Guide: Written By and For Lesbian Women* will hopefully be a handbook that every lesbian woman or couple interested in creating a family will have on their bookshelves.

The sharing of resources from one lesbian to another is paramount to our community's connectedness. In this book, we seek to connect with other lesbian women by sharing the pitfalls and successes we experienced en route to our babies' conceptions. And so, in the chapters to come, we will tell our story. We hope that it will affirm your desire and plans to have a child, and teach you what we wish we had known . . . in the beginning. Best wishes for a smooth, positive donor insemination experience, and a speedy and healthy conception!

Chapter One

A Foundation

If you are reading this book, then you are considering starting a family. This is a very exciting time in your life. However, for women desiring to conceive through donor insemination, the path to conception requires a different road map. Understanding and developing an intimate relationship with the donor insemination process then becomes essential. This book is intended to provide you with a guided tour through the nuts and bolts of the process, helpful tips that may increase your chances of conception, and detailed accounts of *our* insemination experiences, which are presented in order to give life to the concept of donor insemination.

Before we begin our discussion about donor insemination (DI), we first want to appropriately attend to the importance of this monumental decision, to plan for a family. Having a baby signifies a turning point in our lives. Based on my (Marie's) earlier work, *Homosexual Rites of Passage: A Road to Visibility and Validation* (1999), just *making the decision* to plan for a family is a significant rite of passage. It requires an entirely new level of maturity and commitment toward personal growth. Family planning is part of a larger life-enhancing journey, and it is an awesome commitment. It is clearly one of the most important decisions that women can make. Lacy and I discussed our desire to have a baby for seven years before we actually made the commitment to actively plan our baby's conception. Everyone has her own timetable and her own rate of growth. What is important to highlight at this juncture is that *making the decision* to plan for a family and to parent is a very exciting rite of passage in the lives of lesbian women, because it marks the beginning of an incredible journey that in years past may have seemed impossible!

1

Based on our experiences, we found the journey toward parenthood can be broken down into three distinct stages. The first stage involves the aforementioned *making the decision* to plan a family and parent, the second involves committing to and *implementing the inseminations* to achieve conception, and the third and lengthiest stage includes *pregnancy, giving birth, and child rearing.* If we think of rites of passage as transitions in our lives that mark significant personal growth experiences and development, then each stage that lesbians face en route to achieving parenthood through donor insemination is a significant rite of passage. And thus, these stages that facilitate growth not only are critical to the short-term goal of conceiving a child, but also enhance us as people by strengthening our sense of character and giving life to the expressions "unconditional love" and "self-sacrifice."

Having been through this process ourselves, we suggest that you maximize your personalization of our message by maintaining an open mind and permitting full absorption of the presented material. As you read each chapter, continue to explore your feelings about each component in the process. Recognize, explore, and grow to understand your fears, frustrations, hopes, dreams, desires, uncertainties, obstacles, solutions, personal growth and development, and feelings of utter joy and excitement. By allowing the full range of these experiences into your life, you will find yourself gaining the necessary strength that will aid your ability to succeed in this process, and ultimately to raise a whole, tolerant, intellectually and emotionally intelligent child.

We can certainly attest to the fact that we experienced quite a range of emotions throughout the donor insemination process. Initially, we felt a great deal of excitement as we shared our dreams with each other. That was quickly followed by frustration, fear, and impatience, as we realized and experienced the many obstacles that can impede conception. At times, we even (fleetingly) contemplated giving up; however, we always chose to "get back in the saddle again." It is our goal in this book, first and foremost, to validate lesbians' experience of intense emotions throughout this process so that others do not feel alone in their journey. In addition, we want to provide a definition and description of the donor insemination process, a discussion of potential pitfalls, issues, and helpful tips in the context of "what the doctors don't often tell you," and then a description of our experiences with each component in the process. We want this book to act as a shared resource, so that lesbian women trying to create families through donor insemination can be confident, informed consumers.

With that in mind, let us share with you an overview of *our* journey, to invite you into the world of donor insemination. We began this process quite methodically, rationally, and optimistically. When making plans for our baby's conception, we fully enjoyed romanticizing the notion of having a baby together. For us, these baby plans represented the ultimate consummation of our union. We were very happy and excited to fantasize about raising our baby together, in a home full of love and nurturance. We talked about our baby-to-be as a creation of love, and we indulged many visions of our baby's room, full of colorful toys and playful noise. We shared our wonderment about the traits the child would bring into the world and the traits that he or she would learn from each of us. We thoroughly enjoyed living, breathing, and dreaming in this bubble of our imaginations. (And rightly so, because these dreams are what give us the strength to pursue the path to parenthood!)

However, our romantic notions were quickly thwarted when we realized that the actual process of conceiving through donor insemination is not romantic at all. In fact, it is quite medically technical, often taking place in a sterile environment. Such a realization facilitated a temporary shift in our thinking from "having a baby" to enduring a medical procedure in order to become parents. While disconcerting at times, this mental shift was crucial to understanding the scope of our endeavor. We quickly learned that this more technical viewpoint led to the need to become educated consumers and play a more active role in our attempts at conception. Thus, while our enthusiastic and romantic baby dreams were very much a part of our drive to continue with the insemination process, the reality of the medical nature of the donor insemination process required an acceptance that having a child would require knowledge, patience, financial resources, and love.

Perhaps the largest unexpected obstacle we faced throughout the process was the emotional turmoil associated with fertility issues. Our relationship strength combined with our ability to communicate, as well as having a basic understanding of the process, perhaps gave us a false sense of emotional security and preparedness. Our first few months of inseminations taught us just how emotionally *un*prepared we were. Ultimately, the intense roller coaster of emotions became the most stressful element in the process for us, outweighing any of the financial burdens and/or the stress of the inseminations themselves. This emotional stress was a result of a number of issues that will be described throughout this book.

Another obstacle we faced was the scarcity of available resources on donor insemination–specifically, resources that addressed issues pertaining to the lesbian minority. In the areas of gay and lesbian studies as well as infertility/health sections of many bookstores, increasing numbers of books about male/female infertility, child development, and parenting can be found. But many of these resources do not specifically describe and validate the trials and tribulations that lesbian women experience en route to successful conception via donor insemination. For instance, Clunis and Green's (1995) *The Lesbian Parenting Book: A Guide to Creating Families and Raising Children* and Noble's (1987) *Having Your Baby by Donor Insemination: A Complete Resource Guide* are two examples of currently available resources. Clunis and Green's work addresses child development, potential lesbian parenting dilemmas/issues throughout the developmental years, and possible ways to deal with particular issues from a lesbian perspective. Noble's work provides a thorough description of the donor insemination process, including the "how-to's," the pros and cons of different procedures, and the pros and cons of known and unknown donors. However, there are limits to these authors' works with respect to their role as resources for *lesbian* women desiring to *become* parents. Clunis and Green devote only one chapter to the issue of creating families through donor insemination, while the remainder of the work emphasizes the stages of lesbian parenthood and child development. Noble's work provides a thorough description of the donor insemination process, but it was not written to address the issues specific to lesbian women. In our opinion, it is biased against the use of unknown donors, some information is outdated, and it addresses a number of male infertility issues which are not relevant to lesbian women. In addition to the limited amount of available resources for the lesbian community on this subject, some of the literature that is available was found to present conflicting information when resources were compared. Given the small window of time during her cycle when a woman can successfully conceive (which will be described further in later chapters), lesbian women *literally* cannot afford to be uneducated consumers with inaccurate or inconsistent information.

Another unexpected obstacle that we faced was doctor insensitivity, inconsistency, and incompetence related to donor insemination. Given the critical timing and technique involved in the donor insemination procedure, it is essential for lesbian women to feel confident that their health care practitioner is supportive of lesbian women, thoroughly knowledgeable about and experienced with the insemination process and related fertility issues, and sensitive to and respectful of individual patient needs. The health care practitioner should be a stress-reducing agent, not a catalyst for stress. We were floored, to say the least, to experience such mistreatment and insensitivity at the hands of a practice of doctors we originally thought to be our allies and "family facilitators."

Lastly, predicting ovulation became a regular challenge each month–a fact that also was not anticipated. Armed with basic information from the literature, we tracked all of my monthly menstrual changes with meticulous detail in order to accurately predict ovulation. Therefore, in the beginning, we felt confident that we had a thorough understanding of my menstrual cycle patterns, and most importantly, my ovulation. However, our lack of supportive, knowledgeable doctors in those early months contributed to our not knowing that a woman can show fertile, regular monthly menstrual cycles and still experience ovulation irregularity. After probing further in the literature on infertility, we discovered that it is very common for doctors who regularly perform inseminations to routinely prescribe a low dose of a fertility medication (even to women with regular menstrual cycles) in an attempt to "control" a woman's ovulation. This is done in an effort to counteract the inherent stress involved in the donor insemination process that so often affects the predictability of ovulation.

We are convinced that our ability to persist in advocating for proper, precise health care was the single most important determinant (secondary to the sperm and egg, of course) in our successful conceptions. Unlike many other medical procedures that can demonstrate accurate cause and effect relationships and that can account for certain types/degrees of error, the medicine and art of donor insemination do not often offer such clarity. The reasons why one insemination results in conception and another does not, in fertile women, often remains a mystery. This is perhaps the most important reason to minimize the chances of human error, through donor insemination education, preconception efforts to create what we call "womb wellness," and positive and clear communications with doctors and donors.

As you read through this resource guide, consider each component in the process as it relates to you. If an issue or procedure that we present remains unclear, please make a commitment to yourself to pursue clarity through additional resources. Remember: knowledge is power, and gaining an understanding of this process facilitates positive thinking and stress reduction. These factors alone can increase a woman's chances of conception. Throughout the remainder of this work, you will read about donor insemination, issues that lesbian women face when undergoing inseminations, sperm, women's menstrual and ovulation cycles, doctor- and donor-assisted inseminations, the preconception period and stress reduction, the issue of known versus unknown donors, family and societal support, and related issues. We hope the topics discussed in our resource guide will validate your experiences and the information provided will assist you in achieving conception and creating your family. It is an exciting opportunity for us to be able to affirm and participate in the lesbian baby boom!

Chapter Two

The Swimmers

Removing the mystery, fear, and uncertainty about donor insemination requires increasing women's knowledge and comprehension of the process. To do this, we must first gather facts and learn a core vocabulary of terms. This allows us to become active participants in our family planning endeavors *from the beginning*. Active participation facilitates empowerment, and this sense of empowerment is a critical component in our lesbian lives and in this process. With the current state of managed care and its demands on doctors, as well as homophobic attitudes in our society, empowerment is essential.

The first step in the information-gathering phase is to define briefly and clearly exactly what donor insemination is all about. Donor insemination is essentially the act of inserting sperm obtained from a known or unknown male donor into a woman's vagina, cervix, or uterus with the intent to conceive a child. The acquisition of the donor sperm will be described in greater depth in later chapters. But, for the purpose of this initial introduction to the terminology, the most common means of collecting sperm for donor insemination (either through a known local donor or through a cryobank) is a male's masturbation and ejaculation into a wide-mouthed clean/sterile container. This is a simplified definition, but the truth is the act of insemination *is* quite simple. However, the challenge of donor insemination rests in the fact that while the *act of insemination* involves the simple placement of sperm into a woman's reproductive organs, the *voyage to conception* is much more intricate. The body's processes that must synchronize at precisely the right moment in order to conceive a child are a key focus in this book.

Millions of members of a swim team, otherwise known as sperm, are critical participants in this synchronization process that makes conception possible. Therefore, in order to address the different types of donor insemination and the many related issues that accompany such an intricate process, it is essential that we first become familiar with the swimmers that contribute a solid fifty percent of our baby's genetic material. The remainder of this chapter will focus on the essential role that sperm plays in conception. Namely, we will address the qualities of sperm that make it viable (capable of fertilizing eggs) and the differences between frozen and fresh sperm.

THE SPERM ITSELF

Understandably, lesbian women in general may not have cause to learn about the male reproductive system and its components. However, lesbian women wishing to inseminate and conceive by donor insemination are catapulted into a new realm of information-seeking and intrigue in this area. Thus, information that previously appeared irrelevant will become important as you broaden your knowledge base.

Bearing that in mind, the literature outlines the advantages and disadvantages of using fresh and frozen sperm–information many doctors neglect to explain. This information will be disseminated later in this chapter. But first, it is important to discuss the characteristics of sperm, whether fresh or frozen.

Several key components make sperm viable, or capable of fertilizing a woman's eggs. The number of sperm (in concentration), the motility of the sperm, the amount of semen, and the shape of the sperm are all essential aspects which help determine the sperm's viability. Before defining each of these qualities of sperm, we want to distinguish between sperm and semen (as the two terms are often used interchangeably and we want to avoid confusion). Semen refers to the fluid that the male donor ejaculates at the time of orgasm. Semen may or may not contain sperm, and it is impossible to determine whether the semen contains sperm simply by looking at it with the naked eye. Sperm can only be detected and counted with the aid of a microscope. They resemble little tadpoles, with a head and a tail. The head contains the donor's genetic material, and the tail whips back and forth to aid in the sperm's locomotion. In a fertile donor, an ejaculate should contain millions of sperm that move at a rapid pace. In summary, the donor's ejaculate, namely semen, is the fluid that *contains* the sperm.

Given that basic description of sperm and semen, let's talk about the important qualities of sperm that make it capable of fertilizing a woman's eggs. The *number of concentrated sperm* is one of the first things to consider. Sperm can be counted by taking a small portion of the male's ejaculate and looking at it in a "counting chamber" under a microscope (Silber, 1980, p. 66). A technician then performs the task of counting each sperm that is located within a certain number of boxes in the counting chamber, which serve to represent a certain amount of fluid. The total number of sperm in the ejaculate is then calculated from that information. If the count is ten million sperm per cc, which is a fairly low count, it means that the technician will have counted ten sperm within five boxes of the counting chamber. If ninety million sperm per cc were determined to be present, a fairly high count, the technician would have counted ninety sperm within five boxes. The "per cc" component of the reading discloses that the number described is the actual numerical sperm concentration per cubic centimeter (Silber, 1980, p. 66).

A second critical characteristic of sperm is the *sperm's motility*, or the sperm's speed and the quality of its movement. In ejaculate, there is always a certain number of mobile and immobile sperm. The immobile sperm obviously are not capable of swimming to and through a woman's cervical mucous and reaching her egg. However, the moving or motile sperm are prepared for this journey and may differ in types of movement. Lab technicians use different grade levels with which to evaluate and calculate the quality of the sperm's movement. The grade levels range from 1-4, with grade one being that the sperm are only able to wiggle lethargically in place with little or no forward progression and grade four being that sperm are capable of moving straight ahead at a very quick rate. Grades three and four are generally capable of fertilizing a woman's eggs, while grades one and two typically are not (Silber, 1980, p. 66).

The *shape of the sperm* is another important characteristic. The structure of the sperm goes hand in hand with the motility of the sperm. Generally speaking, sperm that are abnormally shaped (including sperm that are large, small, two-headed, or with tails that are kinked in some way) demonstrate poor motility, while normal sperm (characterized by having oval-shaped heads and long, straight tails) display good motility.

And, finally, the *volume of semen* that a man ejaculates is a significant component in the fertilization process. An average ejaculate amount is between one-half teaspoon and a full teaspoon. Translated into "cc measurements," this amounts to between 2.5 and 5 cc's (Silber, 1980, p. 67). Silber claims that the number of sperm released into the female's vagina has been found to be less important than the actual concentration of the sperm within the semen. Thus, some males may think they are fertile and producing a lot of sperm because they see a large ejaculate, but they may in fact have a low *concentration* of sperm in that large semen sample. Silber also states that larger ejaculate volumes can result in the sperm getting diluted in the large amount of fluid. Ultimately, bigger is not necessarily better in terms of ejaculate size; it is the concentration of sperm in the semen that is significant.

As illustrated above, the concentration and the quality of the sperm are important factors that often dictate the sperm's ability to fertilize an egg. Thus, it is crucial to understand these qualities of sperm as they relate to the fresh and frozen sperm used in donor insemination.

FRESH SPERM

Fresh sperm can be defined as sperm obtained from fresh ejaculate that is not chemically preserved or altered in any way. Fresh sperm is reported to be *the most viable* type in terms of chances for conception. A fresh sperm sample is generally larger in volume and contains more sperm than what is typically found in a frozen sample. In addition, fresh sperm are more mobile in respect to both speed and quality of movement. Finally, and perhaps most importantly, fresh sperm stay alive and capable of fertilizing an egg in a woman's fallopian tubes for approximately 48 to 72 hours. This is important to know as this fact alone may dictate the point at which you inseminate. We are compelled to mention at this point that medical personnel often disagree with respect to the life span of the sperm; however, we feel confident that 48 to 72 hours is a conservative estimate for fresh sperm based on our review of the literature.

For lesbian women, fresh sperm may be considered a luxury; however, it is not the only option!

FROZEN SPERM

Frozen sperm can be defined as the semen sample that a cryobank (sperm bank) obtains from a registered male donor in their program, which is preserved using a freezing technique, for quarantine and eventual use. The cryobanks report that their registered donors ejaculate the fresh semen sample into a sterile container at the cryobank. The specimen is then mixed with a cryoprotectant buffer (generally, glycerol drops or egg yolk citrate) to aid the semen in surviving the freeze/thaw process. This mixture is then drawn up into a vial and undergoes the freezing process (i.e., being placed in a controlled-rate freezing machine). Once frozen, the specimen is placed into storage at approximately −196 degrees centigrade for a six-month quarantine. (As you can see, freezing sperm should not be tried at home.) At the end of those six months, the donor provides a fresh sample. The fresh sample and the quarantined frozen sample are then retested in order to rule out select infectious diseases before the frozen sample can be released for use (Fairfax Cryobank marketing materials, 1999, pp. 3-4).

When the specimen is purchased and sent to the doctor's office for insemination (it is sent in one of the cryobank's liquid nitrogen shipping tanks which guarantees to keep the sample frozen and viable for a certain number of days from the date of shipment), the vial is then removed from the tank and thawed according to the cryobank's instructions. Typically, a sample can be thawed in a brief amount of time (generally minutes) in one of three ways:

1. Placing the sealed vial in warm water;
2. Leaving the sealed vial on a table at room temperature;
3. Holding the sealed vial in one's hand or placing it next to the skin in some way–holding it under a breast, for example. Body temperature is the key to this method.

Once thawed, the sample should be checked under a microscope by the doctor or by a medical assistant to check the sample's motility. If adequate, the insemination is performed.

FRESH VERSUS FROZEN SPERM–A COMPARISON

The bottom line is that fresh sperm are definitely more viable than frozen sperm. Fresh sperm have greater motility, and they live in a woman's fallopian tubes longer than frozen sperm, which means fewer samples are needed to cover a longer window of a woman's peak fertile time. In 1987, Noble claimed that

> about one third more inseminations are required using frozen semen because it is two thirds as viable as fresh sperm. About 65 percent of sperm survive the freezing technique. . . . Ice crystallization and respiratory shock are the main problems for the sperm with cryopreservation. (p. 115)

In addition, in a newsletter printed by the Sperm Bank of California (Winter, 1999), a staff writer claimed:

[women] are fertile for only 6 to 12 hours during each cycle. . . . Using frozen sperm makes [the precise timing of ovulation] even more important. . . . [F]resh sperm will live for 3 to 5 days within a woman's body while frozen sperm will live for *up to* 24 hours. [In addition, they report that women must realize] most of the information out there about insemination . . . is based on the use and characteristics of fresh sperm. This includes recommendations that your doctor may give you, such as inseminating twice, 48 hours apart. . . . Doctors do not learn FAM [Fertility Awareness Medicine] in medical school. (pp. 1-2)

Fresh Sperm–Advantages and Disadvantages

In addition to *favorable sperm characteristics*, using fresh sperm from a local donor has other advantages. *Sperm is available immediately* without shipping concerns or thawing complications. In addition, *the costs involved are often significantly reduced* (or eliminated) because you do not have to pay an inordinate amount for a sample. (Sperm sale agreements will be covered later.) In short, using a known donor with a fresh sample can decrease your costs considerably and increase your chances of covering your peak days of fertility each month.

Disadvantages for using fresh sperm include the fact that generally *each sample is often not diagnostically tested* in order to rule out transmittable diseases and other genetic disorders. The other significant disadvantages for the use of fresh sperm *relate to legal and emotional ramifications of this process.* Specifically, to use fresh sperm means that the donor lives locally; and it generally means that the donor's identity is known. While this may not be a negative factor in everyone's life, it certainly presents long-term issues one must consider. We feel these long-term issues will weigh out as a disadvantage for some lesbian women. These important issues will be addressed in greater depth later in Chapter Five.

Frozen Sperm–Advantages and Disadvantages

Despite the many advantages of using fresh sperm, a frozen sperm sample is a popular choice for many lesbian women, given the anonymity of the process. Therefore, it is important to know the advantages and disadvantages of using frozen sperm. As mentioned, a major advantage of using frozen semen is that it allows you to select an anonymous donor and purchase his sperm as an *anonymous consumer*. In this day and age, given the many legal issues that coincide with birth parents' rights, it provides a great deal of peace to have the sperm bank act as a third party which permits the identity of the donors and the buyers to remain confidential. Waivers are often signed by all parties accepting or forfeiting rights and responsibilities appropriately.

A second important advantage of frozen sperm is that it is reported to be *carefully screened and quarantined for sexually transmitted diseases and many genetic disorders*. The cryobanks we researched require the prospective donor to be serologically tested for: HIV-1 and HIV-2 antibodies; Hepatitis B surface antigen and core antibody; Hepatitis C antibody; syphilis (or RPR); SGOT and SGPT (these tests detect liver diseases), and HTLV-I (this test detects infection with the human T-cell leukemia virus type I). In addition, semen specimens are tested for chlamydia, mycoplasma, gonococcus, and cytomegalovirus. After the donor's semen samples are quarantined for six months, they are retested for the above listed infectious diseases, including HIV-1, HIV-2, Hepatitis B, and Hepatitis C. Generally, semen cultures are performed every three months, and in some banks, complete serologies on the donor are repeated every three to six months. It is important to note that not all sperm banks necessarily perform all screening tests. Make sure you take the time to research the procedures used, screenings performed, and guarantees offered.

Another advantage of frozen sperm is that it can be *purchased in a "washed" form* (which will be defined and described later in Chapter Four). Essentially, washed semen means that other debris and abnormal sperm have been removed from the sample, which enables the sample to have a concentration of healthy, normal, motile sperm ready for insemination directly into the uterus.

Many lesbian women enjoy and select the frozen sperm option due to their ability to *handpick the characteristics of their donor*. For many couples undergoing donor insemination, it is often appealing for the donor to be selected based on the physical characteristics and personality of the non-biological mother. For single lesbian women, it is empowering simply to have the control and ability to choose desirable donor traits based on individual needs, health histories, and circumstances.

The sperm banks that sell frozen sperm offer the option of purchasing numerous vials of the same donor's semen and storing them at their facility at your expense for later use. Some doctors' offices, however, permit the storage of additional frozen sperm vials at no charge. For some individuals, this provides peace of mind as the same donor can be used repeatedly in subsequent "trials," either monthly or for an additional child. Without an advanced purchase and storage plan, sperm banks normally sell donor vials on a first-come, first-serve basis, based on donor availability at the time of purchase. Thus, we encourage you to plan your inseminations with this in mind, especially if you have your heart set on a particular donor.

A major disadvantage of frozen sperm is the *reduced motility and survivability* due to the freezing process. Thus, even though the frozen sperm are concentrated in the small vial (and we know sperm concentration is a good thing), their reduced motility and shorter life span are definitely issues to consider. Essentially, while fresh sperm can live up to five days, frozen sperm lasts only *up to* twenty-four hours. Thus, either your monthly costs increase when you choose to purchase and use more than one vial of frozen sperm per month in order to increase your odds of conception, or your chances of conception will decrease because of the limits of one sample's lifespan. These are important facts to know and options to consider before purchasing your first month's sample!

Given the facts we know about sperm, a comparison of two large well-known crybobanks' guarantees yielded the following results. The informational packets from the California Cryobank (1998) and the Fairfax Cryobank (1999), two of the larger, nationally known sperm banks, extended different guarantees for the post-thaw quality of their samples and each sample's motility. The California Cryobank stated that each 1 cc intracervical insemination (ICI) vial is "guaranteed to contain a minimum of 20 million (+/−10%) motile sperm after thawing" (California Cryobank marketing materials, 1998, p. 5). Each intrauterine insemination specimen (IUI) packaged in .5 cc vials is "guaranteed to contain a minimum of 12 million (+/−10%) motile sperm (24 million/ml) after thawing" (California Cryobank marketing materials, 1998, p. 5). The California Cryobank's guarantee of motility included a post-thaw minimum motility of 25% for ICI, and 35% motility for IUI (p. 5). The Fairfax Cryobank guaranteed a "minimum quality guarantee of 35% motility and 20 million total motile cells/ml" for both ICI and IUI samples (Fairfax Cryobank marketing materials, 1999, p. 6). If we know that a sperm count of 50 million is average and that a 100 million sperm count is relatively high, then a 20 million or less sperm count is relatively low. In addition, if we know that fifty percent motility is average, then we know that twenty-five to thirty-five percent guaranteed post-thaw motility is on the low end of average. Thus, a *frozen sperm sample is smaller in volume* and *contains less motile sperm than an average fresh sperm sample or even a larger frozen sample.*

Several other disadvantages of using frozen sperm are *the cost, the potential for human error, and complicated "timing" issues.* Frozen semen is generally more costly than fresh sperm, unless you have an entrepreneurial known donor. One ICI vial, on average (at the time this book was written), is priced between $115 and $175, and one IUI vial is priced between $180 and $220. (These costs do not include prices for donors who were doctoral candidates. Their samples generally cost more.) If you purchase two vials per month, the semen samples would generally cost around $400 (based on these estimates). In addition to the purchase price of the semen, there is usually a shipping charge that averages $125. If you inseminate at home, this may eliminate further costs. However, if you are working with a physician, it can easily cost $100 or more for each insemination performed. Overall, it can be quite a financial investment to purchase and inseminate with the samples from a cryobank. We spent an average of $800 per month on the process.

Although it is a disconcerting notion, another disadvantage of using frozen sperm from a cryobank is the possibility of "donor confusion." By "donor confusion," we simply mean that there is a possibility of receiving sperm from a donor you did not choose, whose sample was placed in a vial with your chosen donor's number on it. While the odds of this are slim, this possibility cannot be discounted because of the simple fact that a "middle man" (the sperm bank and its employees) is involved. While the sperm banks make many claims about their efforts to control for human error through coding checkpoints, etc., this risk is something to consider.

Finally, *timing issues with respect to shipping* can exacerbate the anxiety related to the insemination process. Timing your ovulation cycle with the shipping and storage of the samples is crucial, but often stress provoking!

There are no clear right or wrong answers about which type of sperm to use. The information presented in this chapter is provided to facilitate a greater understanding of this process which still may be a bit puzzling to you. Continue to read on, as each chapter builds on and complements the last in order to provide you with a growing sense of empowerment and clarity. We recommend that you allow yourself time simply to be an "information gatherer" at this stage. When the picture feels complete, then weigh out the costs and benefits of each option and detail as it relates to your life, resources, family, needs, goals, and situation.

Chapter Three

Hatching and Catching the Egg

Now that you know more than you ever thought you wanted to know about sperm, we would like to discuss something you are more familiar with: the menstrual cycle. If you are anything like us, you have a basic understanding of your menstrual cycle. Given that most of us get our periods for the first time in early adolescence, we have many years to become familiar with the quirks and patterns of our monthly visitor. In general, women are able to describe their cycles as regular (their period arrives about the same time and has the same cycle length each month) or irregular (there is no consistent pattern with respect to its arrival or departure). We may also have a basic awareness of routine symptoms that present themselves just before our period arrives (typically known as premenstrual syndrome) or symptoms that occur during the initial days of our cycle. And, we can generally predict how long our period will last, perhaps even knowing what kind of flow can be expected on each day. This is all part of being in touch with our bodies and our own personal rhythms. We will ask you in this chapter to prepare to expand this mind-body awareness because it will play an essential role in the planning of your inseminations and the successful conception of your child.

A woman's menstrual period is actually nature's way of indicating that fertilization did not occur during the previous cycle. Just as a male's ability to ejaculate offers no guarantee that there are sperm within the semen, a woman's menstrual period does not guarantee that she is ovulating. The menstrual period, or menses, is but one segment of a full month's cycle. While all phases of a woman's cycle are essential in the process, the phase that we will focus on the most in this chapter is ovulation. Ovulation is defined by Silber (1980) as "the process whereby a mature egg is extruded from the ovary" and then travels through the fallopian tubes to await fertilization (p. 20). While the male reproductive system is largely external, and components of sperm can be fertility-tested rather easily and inexpensively, the female reproductive system (including ovulation processes) is largely internal and requires meticulous monitoring to show signs of fertility and to avoid the high cost and invasiveness of fertility tests. Therefore, we will now focus on the basics of a woman's menstrual cycle and four methods of non-invasively monitoring peak times of fertility.

THE MENSTRUAL CYCLE

Countless books have been written that address the many minute details and components of a woman's menstrual cycle. It cannot be emphasized enough that there is a very crucial biochemical process that occurs within a woman's body prior to and after ovulation that creates an environment in which fertilization is able to take place and the development of a new human being begins. Each and every hormone and structure must synchronize in order to create life and to sustain the developing baby until delivery. Because of the complexities of the human body and, more specifically, the female anatomy, we will leave the medical descriptions to the experts. In doing so, we encourage you to check out the references listed in this book or to find resources that facilitate your comprehension of these miraculous bodily processes. We will, however, describe a few essential details about women's cycles that are pertinent to explaining donor insemination.

Just as Chapter Two covered a core set of terms about sperm in order to promote your active participation in the process, a core vocabulary related to the menstrual cycle will require exploration as well. First and foremost, we will discuss the concept of *cycle length*. It is critical that you know how to count the number of days in your monthly menstrual cycle. Day one of the cycle is considered the first day of bleeding (even if it is only light bleeding). Nofziger (1982) clarifies this further:

> You can tell if the spotting is the real beginning of your period by checking your basal body temperature. If the temperature has started to drop from its elevated phase, then the spotting is the beginning of the period. If the basal temperature remains high during the spotting, and drops the day of the heavier flow, then the day of the increased flow is "day 1" of the cycle (and the period). (p. 80)

Basal temperature charts will be described in greater detail later in this chapter. However, for the purpose of identifying cycle length, upon determining day 1 of your cycle, you count each day of that month until the last day before the next period begins. The total of those days will give you that month's cycle length. For example, if you got your period on October 1, and then got your period again on October 30, you would count a 29-day cycle. You do *not* count the day your period resumes (the 30th, in this case). October 30 would then become day one in the next cycle's count.

Calculating your exact cycle length is crucial to determining retrospectively when ovulation occurred that particular month. *Predicting* ovulation is much trickier than confirming it after if has already occurred. And, in the absence of fertility issues, the ability to *predict* ovulation is the key to getting pregnant. Therefore, understanding your cycle length will assist you in assessing and establishing your fertility patterns and predicting ovulation in the future, and it will also allow you to accurately estimate the date that ovulation occurred in the previous month.

Most women tend to ovulate approximately fourteen days (or two weeks) *before* their next period. Some people may have the misconception (pun intended!) that they ovulate fourteen days *after* they get their period. This error in thinking may be due to the fact that people assume they have a 28-day cycle, and can count fourteen days either way. However, many women do not have perfectly regular 28-day cycles. The experts state that ovulation can occur anywhere between twelve and sixteen days before the next period, which leaves fourteen days as the average. Therefore, if we take our previous example of the October 1 menstrual cycle, counting backwards the fourteen days to confirm ovulation would proceed like this. You take the length of cycle (i.e., 29 days), and subtract 14, which leaves you with the retrospective estimate that the ovulation date was the 15th day of the cycle, or October 15. The 15th day of the cycle was roughly fourteen days before the next period.

Having just covered the basics of how to begin to become aware of your fertility, let us reiterate the short life span of a woman's egg. Women are fertile (capable of having a viable egg available to fuse with a male's sperm) for 12 to 24 hours per month. If the egg is viable for twelve hours, frozen sperm for up to twenty-four hours, and fresh sperm for between forty-eight and seventy-two hours, then the "window" for conception is quite small, and timing becomes everything. Nofziger (1982) illustrates this point:

> [if the follicle] popped at 6:30 A.M. and lived until 7:30 P.M., and you [inseminated] at 10:00 P.M., it would be too late *for that whole cycle.* (p. 21)

Thus, tracking your cycle and confirming ovulation are two measures that are paramount in pinpointing the optimal time of insemination. Because fertility testing for most women can be costly and invasive (unlike testing for men), there are several inexpensive and noninvasive ways to begin to track your body's fertility signs and symptoms. These tracking methods include monitoring your basal body temperature (BBT), cervical mucous (CM), the "Os," and ovulation predictor kit (OPK) test results. Each of these methods will now be defined and described.

BASAL BODY TEMPERATURE (BBT)

Tracking your basal body temperature essentially means that you will be tracking your body-at-rest temperature. Your BBT is a measure of your body temperature after a normal night of restful sleep. It is one of the most natural and most effective ways to track and predict fertility, if used over a period of time. The BBT method monitors natural symptoms within the body that identify different phases of the menstrual cycle, including the days surrounding ovulation.

To track your BBT, you will leave a ready-for-use thermometer on your nightstand that can easily be reached. While past literature asserts that basal, mercury-based thermometers are most accurate, the Center for Disease Control (CDC) currently considers them hazardous waste. Because of this, a name-brand digital thermometer, which also permits temperature readings in single tenths of a degree, may be substituted. Whichever thermometer you use, use it throughout the cycle so that the readings are consistent. The BBT method is most effective when you have had a minimum of "three hours of uninterrupted sleep. . . . [and when] the time [of day] that the temperature is taken [is consistent]" (Noble, 1987, p. 368). At the same time every morning, immediately upon waking and prior to engaging in even the slightest of activities (including getting out of bed), put your thermometer in your mouth under your tongue and remain still in bed for 3-5 minutes. Then remove the thermometer, read your temperature, and record the temperature on a BBT chart (see Appendix A). Before discussing how to fill out the BBT chart properly, it is necessary to describe how the BBT works, what it tells you, and a limitation of the method.

If we know that our BBT is our body at rest temperature, and if our internal biochemical processes are working properly, women often show a routine pattern on their temperature charts. This pattern should demonstrate that in the days *prior* to ovulation, basal body temperatures are always lower than the temperatures taken *after* ovulation (Silber, 1980, p. 89). Noble (1987) claims that this rise in temperature is generally "three to six tenths of a degree" (p. 368); while Silber claims that it is generally a "one degree Fahrenheit" shift (p. 89). The hormone progesterone, secreted in a woman's body by the corpus luteum *only after* ovulation, is what raises her BBT (Silber, 1980, p. 89). It is the progesterone-induced rise in tempera-

ture that we are measuring. When movement from low to high temperatures can be established as a relatively routine pattern across several cycles,
then a woman may be more confident in predicting the time of ovulation.
The BBT monitoring should be done for two to three cycles *before* you begin inseminations in order to give you a baseline of your fluctuations in cycle and the predictability of your ovulation. Silber claims that the BBT is
"the most accurate method of determining ovulation" (p. 89). While this
may be true, a limitation of the BBT is that it only serves to confirm ovulation *after* it occurred that particular month. However, despite this fact, this
method can provide other helpful information about a woman's fertility if
her charts (for a period of three months or more) are viewed simultaneously and particular patterns can be identified. These patterns can facilitate an overall understanding of peak days of fertility, and essentially rule
in particular days in the cycle that a woman is likely to ovulate.

The one potential problem with the BBT method involves human error.
If a woman's temperature is not taken first thing in the morning (before any
activity takes place, which includes getting up and searching for the thermometer), the thermometer reading may be elevated and distort that day's
results. Even small activity levels can raise the BBT from an at-rest reading,
and produce false and unusable results. It is the pattern of daily temperatures over the course of the month that provides the most information. If
the recorded temperatures are inaccurate, the chart is worthless.

Recording the daily temperatures on a chart may not be as easy as you
think. The chart permits you to mark the days of your menstrual period,
days of insemination, days of the cycle and dates of the month, daily temperatures, medications taken, and other cycle observations. Fill in the
dates of your month's cycle, with day 1 corresponding with the date of
your first day of bleeding. You will take your temperature each and every
day of your cycle as instructed previously, beginning with day 1 of your period, in the morning before getting out of bed or engaging in any activity.
After your temperature is taken, you will score the temperature on the
chart in the appropriate day and date column. Place an "X" in the appro-

priate boxes on the chart for the days that you menstruate. In addition, place an "X" in the "insemination box" for the days that you inseminate, and an "X" in the appropriate boxes if you take any medication (especially fertility medication). When you get your next month's period, total up your cycle length and determine your day of ovulation based on the "counting backward fourteen days" method. Note whether it coincided with a rise in temperature. Circle the date of your next period, and then begin another chart with the date of your period becoming day 1 of the next cycle. After you take your temperature each day, and then record the information on the chart, you can then move on with your daily routines. Each evening, double check to make sure that the thermometer is ready for use in the morning and that it is placed in your easy-to-reach spot on your nightstand.

Reading and interpreting your cycle chart is crucial. Therefore, it is very important to be accurate and thorough when recording temperatures *and* recording notes about anything that may have affected your temperature on a particular day. For example, it is important to note on your chart if you are sick, stressed, or not getting adequate sleep. These factors can influence temperature readings, and, if they are noted on the chart, they can help discount an uncharacteristic, wacky reading.

When interpreting the peaks and valleys of temperature change, it is very important to note that not all women will show the abrupt, one-day, characteristic rise suggestive of ovulation. Some women may show a more gradual rise over a period of two to three days, while some women may even show an anovulatory cycle (one in which ovulation did not occur) (Noble, 1987, p. 368). What you are looking for on your BBT chart is a rise in temperature that either occurs on one particular day, or occurs in a sort of "stair-step" fashion over a period of a few days. Once you see the rise, you look for your temperature to remain high for the remainder of the cycle. Once your temperature has remained high for three days *after* the shift in temperature, you can assume ovulation has taken place. In terms of the possibility of anovulation, Noble claims that it is normal for women to periodically have menstrual cycles without ovulation, "especially if there is the stress of monitoring them" (p. 368). However, if this happens several times or becomes a pattern, a consult with your doctor may be in order to discuss fertility concerns and workups.

Lastly, it is interesting to note that while there is a characteristic rise in temperature at the time of ovulation that can be seen on BBT charts, there is also a characteristic drop in temperature at the end of the cycle just before a woman's period arrives, if she is not pregnant. If a woman *is* pregnant, her temperature will remain high, well beyond the dates of her expected period.

Because all women do not have regular cycle lengths or consistent patterns of temperature readings, predicting ovulation may be even more challenging and a fertility consultation may be warranted.

CERVICAL MUCUS (CM)

Cervical mucus is essentially the substance or secretion that many women probably think of as their normal monthly discharge. Many women may view this mucus as inconvenient, unaware of its role as a sign of fertility. Cervical mucus "is produced by special cells up inside the cervix and [it] changes character during the monthly cycle" (Nofziger, 1992, p. 30). The changes in the mucosal quality and quantity over the course of the menstrual cycle are key indicators of the stage of fertility. Similar to changes in basal body temperatures, a woman's cervical mucus and its cyclical texture changes are regulated by her reproductive hormones. In the early and latter days of a woman's monthly menstrual cycle, her estrogen levels are low. These low levels of estrogen result in decreased amounts of mucus. At this early point in the cycle, there is essentially no flow of discharge (and most likely, there are no underwear stains). Women do not tend to experience any sensations of wetness, lubrication, or discharge during this time. As a woman's menstrual period ends, her estrogen levels gradually increase in order to prepare her system for ovulation. As the estrogen levels increase, the quantity of her cervical mucus increases. And, as the quantity of mucus builds, the texture of the cervical mucus changes as well (Nofziger, 1992, p. 31).

Nofziger (1992) provides a thorough description of the cyclical changes detectable in cervical mucus (pp. 29-31). Not only will you be *looking* for these monthly changes, but you will be *touching* the mucus for tactile changes in its texture as well (this is all part of heightening your mind-body connection, which is essential to ovulation attunement). Nofziger claims that women often notice the signs of "early mucus" (indicative of slight fertility) when they detect a milky, sticky, pasty, or thick discharge that is often opaque white or yellow in coloring. When you touch this early mucus, it sticks to your fingers like a paste. As estrogen levels continue to rise, the cervical mucus transitions into a "wet fertile" phase. At this point, women may notice that their cervical mucus is changing from sticky and milky (signs of early, slightly fertile mucus) to thin and watery (much more fertile). The mucus increases in quantity, and it becomes clearer. When you put this wet fertile type of mucus between your thumb and index finger to test its texture and consistency, it feels slippery or wet but not stretchy. The mucus is making the transition into a form that helps and nourishes sperm. When a woman's estrogen levels peak, just before she ovulates, her cervical mucus often becomes a stretchy, slick substance that can actually be stretched between the thumb and forefinger in one strand before breaking. This special stretchy quality is called "Spinnbarkeit." Nofziger calls it "Spinn" for short and points out that it indicates the most fertile phase (p. 35). The day in your cycle in which Spinn is detected is likely the day before or the day of ovulation. After ovulation's fertile phase, the cervical mucus will resume its dry or sticky characteristics.

The presentation of cervical mucus can be different for different women. The important thing is that you closely monitor your mucus for its patterns and irregularities; it is important to be in touch with your cyclical changes. In order to check your cervical mucus, you will want to do several things:

1. Check your mucus in the morning before bathing.

2. A good time to check your mucus is right before or after you use the toilet. Do not check just prior to or after having sex. Your body produces a mucus for lubrication when you are about to have sex, and this differs from cervical mucus.

3. The mucus can be found right at your vaginal opening; Noble (1987) suggests that "only the *external* mucus should be evaluated. . . . [Internal] mucus can confuse the timing [of inseminations] if it is taken from the cervix and examined before it flows to the outside" (p. 370). Therefore, checking for vaginal/cervical mucus internally within the vaginal canal is not recommended. Check your *external* mucus discharge that can be found at the opening of the labia.

4. Reach down with your first finger and thumb, and feel the mucus between your fingers. Pay attention to how it looks, and how it feels in your vagina; assess its consistency. Determine if it has any Spinn qualities; see if it is able to be stretched. Record your findings on your BBT chart for that day in the cycle.

5. Begin tracking your cervical mucus immediately after your period ends each month. Check your mucus several times per day during your fertile time.

In general, women tend to see a significant increase in their cervical mucus from the initial dry phase to the early slightly fertile phase to the fertile phase and then to the extremely fertile phase. But that is not *always* the case. Women should focus on the qualities of the mucus, more so than the quantity. Nofziger (1992) reports that there are women who never see or experience the extremely fertile mucus (p. 36). Some women show a gradual increase of the fertile types of mucus as described previously, and some women experience only a small amount of creamy wetness and then feel dry after they ovulate.

While examining your cervical mucus on a daily basis may seem uncomfortable or distasteful, remember that you must get to know your body, its cycles, and its patterns so that you can identify what is normal and what is irregular. Additionally, use two or more tracking methods together in order to increase your chances of successful ovulation prediction. No one method is foolproof.

THE CERVICAL "OS"

In addition to tracking temperatures and cervical mucus, there are also changes that occur to the cervix itself that indicate fertility. This method of tracking your body's changes is optional, but it may be helpful to those who are interested. Let's take a moment and review the structure of the cervix.

The cervix is essentially the opening into the uterus. It is the

> narrow, lower part of the uterus that fits into the top of the vaginal canal and produces fertile mucus when the hormone estrogen is high. (Nofziger, 1992, p. 87)

The opening to the cervix is called the "Os." As estrogen levels rise and fall throughout a woman's monthly cycle, several corresponding cervical changes occur. The physical changes that can often be detected include: a change in the height and tilt of the cervix (and entire uterus), the firmness of the cervix (ranging from soft to hard), and the gradual opening of the cervical Os. Each of these changes will be described so you will know what to look for, and then the how-to's of self-examination will be explained.

Throughout the early, infertile days of a woman's cycle, the cervix is typically found low in the vaginal canal tilting slightly toward the back of the vagina. It is at this point in the cycle that the cervix can easily be reached. As a woman's fertile phase draws near, around the time of ovulation, her cervix elevates higher and becomes straighter in the vaginal canal. At this point, her cervix is more difficult to reach. The shift in the cervix's positioning often corresponds with the woman's ability to detect cervical mucus at the vaginal opening or on her underwear (Nofziger, 1992, pp. 88-89). Lauersen and Bouchez (1991) claim that the change in the positioning of the cervix "places the opening in a better position for sperm passage" (p. 199). The change in the cervix's elevation is one clue that indicates your body is preparing for ovulation.

Another cervical indicator of impending ovulation is the softening of the cervix. After ovulation and throughout the other infertile phases of the cycle, a woman's cervix will feel rather firm and dry. As the fertile phase begins and the cervix begins to rise, it will also begin to soften. Right before ovulation, a woman can feel her cervix to be wet with fertile mucous, high in her vaginal canal, and soft "like the texture of [her] lips" (Nofziger, 1992, p. 88).

The Os, the cervical opening itself, undergoes changes as well. Nofziger claims that the cervical Os opens over a period of approximately five days (p. 88). During the infertile phases of the monthly cycle, the Os is closed, containing a mucus plug that serves to protect the uterus from infections and other harmful debris. It is during this infertile time that the closed Os will feel like a little dimple that your finger cannot penetrate. As a woman enters the fertile phase of her cycle, awaiting ovulation, the Os will gradually open to enable her to slide a fingertip into the cervical opening about 1/4 to 1/2 of an inch (Nofziger, 1992, p. 88). After ovulation, the Os closes again to protect the uterus until the next fertile phase.

These changes of the cervix are best used to corroborate and confirm the other ovulatory signs (i.e., BBT and cervical mucus). To check the Os and the gradual softening of the cervix, you can:

1. Monitor these changes during your first or second trip to the bathroom in the morning.
2. First, wash your hands, so that even your fingernails are clean.

3. While standing, curl forward a bit, resting one foot on a stool, the toilet, or a chair.

4. Place one or two fingers into your vaginal canal, and reach toward your backbone to find your cervix.

5. Your cervix should feel like the shape of a rubber stopper, or plug.

6. If you have difficulty reaching your cervix, you may have better luck if you press your abdomen down from the outside with your other hand.

7. When you find your cervix, feel for and make note of the positioning of the cervix (whether it is high or low), the size of the Os opening, and the texture of the cervix (whether it is firm and dry or soft and wet).

While tracking the changes in the cervix and Os may help some women to more accurately identify their fertility patterns, it may simply add stress for others. Each woman has to find what is comfortable for her individual needs. We simply recommend using a combination of at least two techniques to track the fertile changes in your cycle. Some women will choose more, and some fewer.

OVULATION PREDICTOR KITS (OPKs)

Ovulation predictor kits provide, generally, a five-day supply of tests which are reported to measure the amount of luteinizing hormone (LH) found in a woman's urine. LH is one of the key hormones that has been identified as critical to ovulation. Ovulation predictor tests are essentially attempting to measure a surge in LH that is found just prior to ovulation. Here is how the test generally works:

1. On the peak days surrounding the window of fertility, a woman is instructed either to urinate directly on a test stick or to urinate into a specimen cup and then transfer a few drops of urine onto the test plate. (The sticks or test plates are treated with a chemical solution.)

2. After approximately three minutes, women are instructed to look for color changes on the test that will indicate the LH levels excreted from their bodies. Generally, the test results are considered "readable" for three to ten minutes after the urine was added, and then the test should be discarded. When reading the test, women are instructed to compare the color of the line in the control window to the color of the line in the test window. When the color of the test line is the *same as or darker than* the color of the control line, the manufacturers of the ovulation predictor kits claim that that is a positive test reading. A positive reading predicts that a woman will ovulate *within* the next 24-48 hours.

3. The color of the test line ranges from very light or light (which indicate lower levels of LH found to be present) to the same color as the control line (indicating elevated LH levels) to very dark (indicating peak LH levels).

4. Women are then instructed to make love or inseminate within 12 to 24 hours after their urine test darkens or shows a positive result (Lauersen and Bouchez, 1991, pp. 200-201).

Because of the critical timing involved in predicting ovulation for donor insemination, the option of using an ovulation predictor kit offers many women hope. However, while the concepts behind the predictor kits are encouraging, there are several limitations that should be highlighted. Lauersen and Bouchez (1991) claim that the onset of menopause can result in raised LH levels, which can create false positives or false readings. They also claim that certain fertility medications can affect the results of ovulation predictor tests. Noble (1987) claims that "rapid LH estimates . . . are not always sufficiently sensitive [when checking] for that hormone peak" (p. 96).

In addition to the limitations presented by the above authors, we encountered several limitations in our own experiences. The most frustrating task for us was reading the test line and evaluating its message. Determining the shade of the line is a subjective observation and assessment, which is always susceptible to human error. It is the *degree* of color that matters most when test lines are compared to control lines. With the small window that lesbian women have to "get it just right," and the expense of sperm samples, shipments, and doctor fees, we found relying solely on a shade of color difference to be extremely stressful.

Another limitation involves the fact that manufacturers recommend taking the test at approximately the same time each day through the peak period, and state that better samples are often collected after 12 noon. Women therefore need to have knowledge of their cycle lengths and "peak periods" to know when to begin testing. And they need to be able to test consistently at the same time each day in that month.

One other limitation is the fact that too many or too few drops of urine placed on the test strip can influence or confound the results, leaving women to feel uncertain about the accuracy of the test. Also, the window of time that women can read the test results creates uncertainty about the accuracy of these tests, because the test and control lines often show different degrees/shades of color beginning at three minutes, and at each progressive minute as the test time approaches ten minutes, at which time the test is considered "over." This leaves women to question: Which was the most accurate reading? At three minutes? At five minutes, or at ten minutes?

It is important to note that the amount of liquid a woman drinks (even within a few hours of performing the test) can influence the results. In addition, conducting the test too early in the day may skew the results (thus the reason why many manufacturers often recommend not using first morning urine) due to heavy concentrations of hormones generally present in first morning urine. Therefore, too much liquid or too little liquid in a woman's body may affect the results.

And lastly, the ovulation predictor tests create an added expense each month. Given the expense of the sperm samples and of the inseminations themselves, this can compound women's financial stress.

While the ovulation predictor test is not error-proof, it can provide valuable information when used in combination with the other prediction/ovulation tracking methods. It is important to be aware of the many things that can influence the outcome of the test and to learn to minimize the role of these factors. We cannot emphasize enough that the most effective method of predicting ovulation is a combination of all the methods described above.

OUR STORY

After several cycles of trial and error and continuous research into the matter, Lacy and I finally found ourselves using all four methods (the BBT, cervical mucus, the Os, and ovulation predictor kits) to assist our prediction of ovulation. Although these methods did not always synchronize on the day of ovulation, they certainly helped us identify certain rhythms and patterns in my ovulation cycles.

The basal body temperature tracking method was most helpful, as I demonstrated fairly regular and consistent patterns across cycles. However, it took some time to fully understand and interpret my graphs. During the initial months of temperature tracking (before we even began to inseminate), my temperature rose a characteristic half of a degree and remained high at mid-cycle, indicating to us that I had ovulated. However, once we began to inseminate and the stress of the process took its toll, I began to show the rise early in my cycle or late in my cycle, and it did not appear to follow the original predictable pattern that we had first seen. This was frustrating! Just when we thought we had it down, the pattern would change.

Because we did not have a sensitive, communicative doctor with whom we could discuss these issues, and the doctors did not assist us in understanding the terminology, we (in perfect hindsight) can say that we sometimes employed an inaccurate vocabulary to describe our experiences. To give you an example, we would explain to the different doctors that my menstrual cycles were regular, but that we could not "catch" ovulation. Our self-report of this experience was never addressed. It is clear that what we needed to communicate, *or what the doctors should have asked about and discussed with us*, was that my temperature charts began to show *irregular ovulation cycles* while maintaining relatively regular cycle lengths. The stress of the tracking procedures, working with insensitive doctors, and the uncertainty of fertility all contributed to throwing my "time of ovulation" out of whack. The BBT charts clearly indicated this phenomenon, and it would have been helpful had our physicians been willing to take a look at our charts. We simply lacked the vocabulary of terms and self-assurance during those initial months of inseminations to assert and describe the irregularity of my ovulation cycles. For many of you who may be using the BBT charts, and who are reading this book to familiarize yourself with core terms and concepts that are essential in this process, the BBT chart *is* extremely valuable when the charts are accurately tracked. We do not doubt the accuracy of our charts; we simply did not employ doctors who were willing or able to interpret them properly.

As for cervical mucus, I generally progressed through Nofziger's identified mucosal phases in textbook fashion. I would experience the dry phase right after my period, and then make the transition into the early fertile mucous stage. I then would see wet, fertile mucus for one to two days, before I would experience the extremely fertile phase and its characteristic Spinn. Of course, this was all documented on my temperature chart, which made it easy to recognize patterns over time. The rise in temperature (indicating ovulation had occurred) coincided with the cessation of cervical mucous. Therefore, most of the time, my temperature and the mucous records would complement each other.

As for the Os, initially we did not track the Os changes every month. However, as we became more educated about this method, we employed it more often in the latter months. I definitely could track the opening and straightening of the cervix and cervical Os prior to ovulation, as well as the closing and drying up period after ovulation. Unfortunately, this did not always coincide on the same day that my Spinn ceased and my temperature rose, leaving us confused at times. Our experience in tracking the changes of the Os was that it provided helpful *supplemental* information, but it was not as reliable in tracking my cyclical changes as the BBT and the cervical mucous methods.

Lacy and I both have mixed feelings about ovulation predictor kits. While they were our greatest source of angst, they were the ultimately the reason we conceived our sons. Perhaps the most anxiety-provoking characteristic of these tests is the fact that you must subjectively compare shades of color to determine the test outcome. Believe me, when you know that you are supposed to ovulate on a given day and you want nothing more in the world than to get pregnant, those test lines become pretty blurry! Lacy and I spent many indecisive moments together agonizing over whether or not a test line was "the same as or darker than" the control line. Furthermore, we discovered over a period of time (and after a significant amount of money) that different brands of the kits showed different results with varying degrees of accuracy. In addition, we found that I demonstrated high levels of LH in the *early, mid-, and late morning*, regardless of when I drank, ate, and urinated. Because of these elevated LH readings in the morning often resulting in a false positive, and our doctor-encouraged reliance on tests to determine whether to inseminate, we felt we were making decisions based solely on a guess. When comparing the results of the ovulation tests with my BBT graphs, cervical mucus notes, and my length of cycle *retrospectively* at the end of each month, we found that I frequently tested positive with the ovulation predictor kits too early in my cycle, with an early insemination the consequence. During the latter months, we began testing in the early afternoon with more credible results.

Ovulation predictor tests are designed to reduce the stress of predicting ovulation; however, our initial experience was that these kits increased the stress and uncertainty involved in this process. Testing later in the day provided better, more accurate test results. Once again, through trial and error, we found our way and discovered how to make the process work.

In the end, in order to control ovulation and counteract the stress of the process, we relied on a low dose of a fertility medication called Clomid (or Clomiphene–consult with your doctor for additional information). Clomid is designed to force a woman to ovulate around days fourteen to sixteen of her cycle with a fair degree of certainty (in the absence of other fertility issues). And for me, Clomid did just that. When paired with Clomid, my BBT charts and patterns, cervical mucus, ovulation predictor tests, and the Os changes served to verify that the predictable changes surrounding ovulation did actually occur. The combination of all of these factors led to our successful conception. We continue to weigh, equally, the importance of fertility medication, the ovulation predictor test results, my BBT patterns, my cervical mucus, and the Os changes.

All women have to find what works for them. Different methods work more reliably for some women than for others. Whichever method or methods you choose, make sure you are tracking them appropriately and accurately. And if you are dealing with the expense and timing of frozen semen at a physician's office, make sure that your doctors are knowledgeable about the process and that they are aware of how you are monitoring your ovulation prediction. Communication is key. In the early months, our inexperience with appropriate language and our lack of confidence in communicating our needs clearly increased our stress related to the process. We hope this book will give you the language we lacked in the beginning, and the knowledge and encouragement to tell your doctor what you need. It is an essential ingredient to your having a positive conception experience!

Chapter Four

Three Types of Donor Insemination

Silber (1980) has created a wonderful framework with which to view donor insemination. In his book *How to Get Pregnant*, he conceptualizes donor insemination as "adopting sperm." He analogizes infertile couples adopting children to fertile females with infertile partners adopting sperm. Just as many infertile couples adopt children to create a loving family environment, lesbian women undergoing donor insemination are adopting sperm to create their families. As adoption has become an increasingly endorsed option in society for creating families, we found this view of donor insemination to be very positive and affirming. Thinking and living in these terms can allow our beliefs about donor insemination to feel more familial. It also provides a wonderful framework through which we can explain this process to our children conceived through donor insemination.

As we ponder the notion of adopting sperm to create family, it is evident that the sperm and a woman's reproductive system each contribute significantly to the ability to conceive children. Each system is responsible for performing fifty percent of the work. This chapter will focus on the procedures that are performed in an effort to unite and fuse these two life-giving systems. Namely, intravaginal inseminations (IVI), intracervical inseminations (ICI), and intrauterine inseminations (IUI) will be addressed. In vitro fertilization (IVF) and other advanced assisted-reproduction techniques are outside the range of our experiences and research, and, therefore, they will not be addressed in this work.

INTRAVAGINAL INSEMINATION (IVI)

For this type of insemination, a woman typically lies on her back (with her hips elevated) while the sperm, whether fresh or thawed, is simply placed inside her vagina by means of a syringe. The syringe must have the ability to draw the sperm in from their storage container, and then to eject the sperm sample into the vagina or vaginal canal. This means of insemination is perhaps most akin to heterosexual intercourse, which achieves the same end: depositing sperm into the vaginal canal and allowing nature to take its course. This can be done at home, without the aid of a physician. In fact, a woman can do this on her own, as this insemination method simply requires the deposit of the sample inside the vagina versus the cervix or uterus. Thus, this method is the only method which allows a woman the option to inseminate herself. It is important to note that metal applicators, syringes, or containers should not be used to store sperm or inseminate women because metal acts as a spermicide (it kills the sperm!) (Noble, 1987, p. 93).

INTRACERVICAL INSEMINATION (ICI)

Intracervical inseminations can be performed privately at home by the parents-to-be, by a supportive DI coach, or by a physician. However, *a speculum is required* for ICI, as it is inserted into the vagina in order to open the vaginal canal and expose the cervix. Therefore, lesbian women choosing to inseminate at home via ICI will need a partner or coach to perform the insemination. Single lesbians who do not have a coach, or who are uncomfortable having their coach perform the procedure, will need a physician.

Intracervical inseminations introduce the sperm, thawed or fresh, slowly around the opening of the cervix (the Os) using a catheter (a syringe with a long narrow tip that can be directed through the vaginal canal up to the cervix opening). This gives the sperm a head start, due to their being placed higher in the woman's reproductive system. The sperm then do not have to swim as long or as far in the acidic vaginal environment (which is one of the first obstacles sperm normally face). By being placed at and slightly into the opening of the cervix, the sperm have bypassed one of their first hurdles. It should be noted that sperm are not placed through the cervix with ICI, for reasons that will be described in the following section.

INTRAUTERINE INSEMINATION (IUI)

Intrauterine inseminations can only be performed by a physician or health practitioner. This procedure utilizes only "washed" sperm, which involves an intricate process completed by a trained professional. Semen samples are washed for IUI using a four-step procedure (Lauersen and Bouchez, 1991, p. 280).

1. The sperm sample is set in a container and left to liquefy at room temperature for approximately thirty minutes.
2. The sperm sample is then mixed with a "culture medium" (that Lauersen and Bouchez describe as akin to fluid which is found inside a woman's fallopian tubes). Once this initial mixing takes place, the sample is then placed into a machine called a centrifuge. The centrifuge spins the sperm, and ultimately separates the sperm from the seminal plasma.
3. After ten minutes, the sperm take the shape of a "small concentrated pellet" that sinks to the bottom (p. 280). This washing procedure can be duplicated up to three times if the sperm sample requires such cleansing.
4. If the sperm count is adequate, the sperm sample is ready at this point for intrauterine insemination (p. 280).

The washing procedure is essential for the sperm to be introduced directly into the uterus. When a woman conceives through sexual intercourse, intravaginal insemination, or intracervical insemination, her cervical mucus (mucus that is produced by and found inside the cervix) plays the vital role of transporting and washing the sperm. Thus, with sexual intercourse,

IVI, and ICI, the cervical mucus is responsible for separating the sperm from other unnecessary or harmful materials found in semen, such as white blood cells, bacteria, dead or abnormal sperm, and prostaglandins (Lauersen and Bouchez, 1991, p. 280). However, during IUI, the sperm bypass the cervix and cervical mucus when they are placed directly into the uterus. This creates the need to "wash" the semen sample (to accomplish what the cervical mucus would do naturally).

Once the sperm are washed, the healthy, uterine-prepped sperm are then drawn up into a syringe with a very long, narrow tip. The woman lies on her back on the examining table, with her feet in stirrups, and the health practitioner then opens the woman's vaginal canal with a speculum, in order to expose her cervix. Once the cervix and, ultimately, the Os are exposed, the health practitioner then inserts the tip of the syringe into and through the Os of the cervix and continues into the uterus. The sperm sample should then be introduced slowly into the uterus to allow the sperm to swim toward the fallopian tubes and then to swim to search for the egg. The reason for the practitioner's introducing the sperm slowly is to prevent uterine cramping, which can be painful for some women. In addition, the cramping caused by introducing the sperm too quickly into the uterus can serve to expel the sperm from the uterus and vaginal canal prematurely.

Lauersen and Bouchez (1991) claim that intrauterine inseminations are "by far the most successful type" (p. 280). In addition, they claim that even though intravaginal and intracervical inseminations do not require washed sperm, washing all sperm samples prior to inseminating aids in increasing a woman's chances of successful conception because washing sperm permits only the "healthiest, most motile sperm to be used for the insemination" (p. 281).

The insemination process, regardless of the type, can be a costly, uncomfortable, and "unsexy" procedure. Many women choose to inseminate at home with the aid of their partner or coach using intravaginal or intracervical methods. In general, at-home inseminations are cheaper and more comfortable, eliminating the need for a physician and his/her sterile office environment. However, it has been our experience that these meth-ods are largely unreliable and anxiety provoking. Therefore, although IUI may appear initially to be the most costly method, spending the money up front on the more successful IUI method may increase chances of conceiv-ing in fewer cycles, saving money over the long haul. We recommend be-ginning with the IUI procedure right off the bat. Our experiences with each type of insemination are outlined below.

OUR STORY

Our first experience with donor insemination began with ICI. The ob-gyn practice that we initially selected would *only* perform intracervical insemi-nations, and we assumed that this method would be effective. We also as-sumed that this medical practice was knowledgeable and competent in the area of donor insemination, given that they advertised it as a specialty in our local pink pages (a telephone book with listings of gay/lesbian or gay/lesbian-friendly businesses). We later discovered that our assumptions were inaccurate. We will expand on our interpersonal experiences with this practice of doctors later in the "Choosing a Doctor" chapter, but it is impor-tant to note at this point that our initial pursuit of ICI (versus other alterna-tives) was simply based on our doctor's recommendation.

I was inseminated at the doctor's office twice a month via ICI for six months, without success. This lack of success–with 20/20 hindsight, of course–was due to a whole host of reasons. Some of these reasons will be presented in order to validate some of your experiences and/or to provide a checklist of things to look out for when you search to select your service provider.

First of all, we were never informed by any doctor in the practice about the differences between fresh and frozen sperm with respect to viability, motility, and life span. It was not until we began to do our own research and ask the doctors the "right" questions that we realized their lack of ex-pertise in this area. We continuously received conflicting information about how long the sperm and egg are viable, as well as issues concerning how many inseminations should be performed in a cycle. Most of the doctors professed that the thawed samples from cryobanks lived up to 72 hours in the woman's system, and, therefore, only one insemination was necessary per cycle. This gave us the impression that the "window for conception" was large, often leading to a great deal of false hope.

In addition to a lack of basic reproductive knowledge, we encountered an abundance of procedural incompetence. Quite often, the physician or nurse practitioner pulled the speculum out too quickly after inseminating, bringing a portion of the already thumbnail-size sample out with it! You can imagine the feeling when I would see $150 to $200 worth of sperm seeping into the paper on the examination table. Topping off such incompetence, the provider would often escort me on my way, without allowing me the twenty minutes of "back time" that is essential to enable the sperm to swim north. Needless to say, the anxiety and frustration we experienced following our first eight to nine cycles with this practice was almost unbearable. Learn from our mistakes: remember to ask your health practitioner to use an appropriately sized speculum, to insert the sample slowly, to remove the speculum slowly, and to leave you on your back (preferably with hips elevated) for at least twenty minutes.

Other common obstacles we faced with this practice were the improper thawing of the sample and the health practitioners' refusal to come into the office for weekend inseminations. We have encountered the common belief that the sample can and should be thawed one to two hours before the insemination, which is *false*. The cryobanks have informed us that a sample should be thawed no more than twenty minutes prior to insemination, as the sperm start dying relatively quickly. Many non-physician, untrained office staff are responsible for the thawing of the sample, so take the time to educate them about this. All of these factors, when looked at collectively, demonstrated the stark reality that the people in this practice did not know what they were doing. Yet, our belief that this practice was one of a kind (serving lesbian couples), combined with our intense hopes of conceiving, compelled us to continue trying despite all of the red flags.

Ultimately, the inconsistent responses we received from the service providers in this practice, combined with their insensitivity and increasingly evident incompetence related to the donor insemination process and procedures, truly deflated our confidence in the practice and in ourselves and my fertility. At this point, our frustrations and pure emotional exhaustion with the medical community led us to revamp our plan and begin at-home IVI inseminations. Firing our doctor and finding a more positive insemination solution gave us a nudge in the direction of reclaiming our sense of empowerment.

With this new sense of empowerment came the belief we could do it all ourselves, cutting out the "middle man" altogether. We tried one month of inseminating at home. We had our cryobank ship our ICI samples directly to our house, and we followed their thawing instructions. We inseminated the ICI samples intravaginally, twenty-four hours apart. This approach to insemination was definitely more positive, and it certainly was more conception-friendly! It was an incredible change to be in the comfort of our own home, in our own bed, and to feel our sense of togetherness and true support of one another. However, it was not to be, as my period arrived on schedule. Once we dealt with the disappointment and emotional let-down, we concluded in hindsight that the issues of an acidic vaginal environment and the natural barrier of my cervical mucus were probably too much for the thawed cryobank sperm to conquer in their less motile state. Although it felt wonderful to inseminate at home and remove the physician as intermediary, we knew we needed to change our plan to increase our chances of conception. It was then that we actively pursued contact with a gay male friend to be our known donor (more on selecting our known donor in Chapter Five).

"T" was our first choice for many reasons, not the least of which was his willingness and open-mindedness. After signing agreements, having him fertility tested, and saving enough money to get to the West Coast (where he lived), we spent ten days inseminating with huge volumes of fresh sperm. T was an amazing sport that month, providing abundant semen samples about every twenty-four hours! Lacy and I (and our donor) felt a surge of confidence that we had, possibly for the first time in our many months of trying, covered the window of my ovulation with virile swimmers. In addition, we inseminated intravaginally each night before I went to bed, allowing the sperm ample time to swim to their destination without the issue of "speculum/sperm fall out." This is why, even to this day, I cannot express completely how disappointing it was to get my period two weeks later. Our commitment to our child-to-be at that point, as well as our emotional resilience, was truly tested. However, we again renewed our commitment to continue our pursuit of creating our family. We regrouped and formulated a new plan.

Upon our return from our unsuccessful venture on the West Coast, we began to discuss the option of IUI. Of course we rationalized that my vaginal secretions were killing the sperm before they could reach the cervix. Therefore, we determined that we must bypass the vaginal canal altogether. Our new "get pregnant at all costs" attitude led us to not only IUI inseminations but fertility medication as well.

The first month, I underwent two intrauterine inseminations, twenty-four hours apart (and notably *none* of the sample leaked out prematurely). In addition, a doctor within the practice ordered blood work for me to verify that I had in fact ovulated. This blood work was to serve as a baseline so that fertility medication could be prescribed the following month. My period arrived roughly two weeks later, and we immediately picked up my prescription for Clomid. Our hopes were high, boosted by a compassionate, competent practice and the help of fertility medication.

I took Clomid as instructed, and underwent two more intrauterine inseminations the next month, twenty-four hours apart. And shockingly, two weeks later, for the first time in thirteen months, my pregnancy test turned positive! We truly felt at that moment the meaning of the old cliché, *the miracle of life!*

Chapter Five

Making the Decision:
Known vs. Unknown Donors

Selecting a donor often marks the transition from the *concept* of donor insemination to the *reality* of the DI process. For some women, their donor decision is an obvious one. For many others, choosing a donor is a journey unto itself. For those who are just beginning the donor selection journey, and for those simply seeking affirmation for a path already chosen, this chapter is devoted to addressing the many issues that can emerge during the donor selection process. We will present several points to consider, aimed at providing greater guidance and clarity for women seeking answers to the emotional, ethical, and legal gray areas that the concept "donor" creates. We will describe these considerations, and then detail our own donor selection experiences.

In Chapter Two we discussed the *physical* characteristics of known and unknown donors' sperm in terms of the *fertility* of frozen and fresh semen. We will now discuss the equally important and powerful emotional and legal issues that are inherent in the donor selection decision.

We believe that many of the emotional issues that surface during donor selection are directly tied to the legal implications of the decision. For many lesbian women, it simply feels safer to purchase samples from unknown donors. This is largely done in order to avoid the possibility of the donor's breaking any agreement and seeking more extensive parental rights. The possibility of a known donor changing his mind about his desired level of involvement is a very real risk and can have serious emotional consequences for both parent(s) and child. It should be noted that some women, particularly single lesbians, may *prefer* a known donor for the very promise of the donor's legal, financial, and parenting involvement. A known male donor who desires to co-parent a child with a lesbian woman or couple may be just what certain lesbian women need to actualize their dream of having a family when a family was previously thought to be an impossibility. In this case, a known male donor may provide not only the sperm needed to create a child, but also the additional support a lesbian woman or couple needs in order to cement the decision to undergo DI. The point we want to make here is to highlight the importance of the potential long-term legal and emotional consequences that co-parenting arrangements may cause. Therefore, we encourage any woman wishing to conceive through known donor insemination to consider this option very carefully. As mental health professionals we realize two things: people have a propensity to change their minds, and we often don't know someone as well as we think!

If the decision is made to use a known donor, please consider legal documentation to "seal the deal" and help in preventing future problems. We recommend that you consider and carefully outline a sperm sale agreement, donor agreement, and parenting agreement. Sample documents and additional information on known donor agreements and issues can be found in the works of Noble (1987), Clunis and Green (1995), and Curry, Clifford, and Leonard (1994). The latter source is *A Legal Guide for Lesbian and Gay Couples*, and it is very helpful regarding these issues and many others. As mentioned, perhaps the most important issue to consider when creating such documents is the extent to which the donor will be involved in the child's life. Will the donor be satisfied with complete termination of all parental rights, including visitation? Or will each party be satisfied with "simple" contacts such as the donor's right to correspond with the child through letters or phone calls? And finally, does everyone agree to a known donor's wanting to parent the child either through visitation, partial custody, or full custody? In the case of women who do want their donors to be involved in their child's life, the donor then is not just a donor . . . the donor is a dad. This option may appeal to some, while it may be out of the question for others. For us, it raised questions about the role of the partner as co-parent, especially concerns over bonding and future conflict for the child. Whatever the decision, make sure that all parties have a complete understanding of the agreement! In the end, you must always remember that even if legal documents are drafted and signed by both parties, their contents can be contested at a later date.

If you choose to rule out the use of a known donor, then the task of selecting your unknown donor begins. We view this selection process as having four phases. These phases include: selecting a cryobank, selecting the type of insemination (ICI/IUI), reviewing donor profiles, and making a selection.

The first phase involves selecting a cryobank from which you will purchase samples and establish an account. For some lesbian women, this will depend on which cryobank your physician works with. Most of the cryobanks that we investigated and considered required a doctor's consent, in which the doctor agrees to supervise the inseminations. Some doctors' offices work exclusively with a specific cryobank, while others will authorize you to do the legwork and select the cryobank that meets your needs. Three well-known sperm banks within the United States are the Fairfax Cryobank in Virginia, the California Cryobank, and the Sperm Bank of California. Of course, there will be others that you will find in your search process, but these three will get you started. (Make sure that the cryobanks you consider are licensed and accredited.) Each will have a slightly different way of doing things, including fee structures, shipping options, issues of doctor consent, donor availability, and availability of donor information. But the end result is the same: they act as a third party, providing semen samples to prospective parents all over the world, permitting anonymity for both the donors and the parents-to-be. We recommend contacting any and all cryobanks and requesting information regarding their services. This information will allow you to make an informed decision that you feel good about!

Phase two of selecting an unknown donor often overlaps phase one. Phase two involves selecting the type of sperm/insemination (ICI or IUI). This was discussed in detail in Chapter Four, and will only be reviewed here in the context of choosing a donor. Oftentimes your physician will have a preference for the type of insemination he or she performs. The medical practice we initially worked with only performed ICI in their office, but they also authorized us to take the samples home and perform the inseminations intravaginally if that was a choice we wanted to make. The second practice we worked with only performed IUI. This dictated the type of sperm we purchased and resulted in in-office inseminations. Ideally, we recommend choosing the type of insemination first and then selecting your doctor (hopefully your ob-gyn will authorize whatever you have chosen). However, this may not be realistic given the area in which you live and doctor availability. Therefore, you may need to be flexible with the resources available in your area. Once you have secured a medical practice and type of insemination, you can begin to shape your donor selection pool (based on ICI/IUI donor availability).

Once the purchase of ICI or IUI vials is clarified, you can then proceed with the third phase of the selection process, reviewing profiles and narrowing down your choices. Having the luxury of choosing and constructing your child's genetic makeup can be a somewhat scary but very exciting process. At times, the information available about a donor may seem overwhelming, while at other times it may seem quite sparse. We found the best way to organize all of the information was to categorize it and then prioritize based on our own beliefs and desires. However, we have learned that women have different priorities when selecting a donor; therefore, our "recipe" as outlined below is meant to be a guideline which we devised after months of having to refine our own process.

1. Most cryobank donor "catalogs" are available free of charge on the Internet or through the mail. This catalog includes: the donor's identification number, race, IUI and ICI availability, blood type, ethnic

background, height, weight, skin tone, eye color, hair color, degree or year in school, and major area of study.

2. The next tier involves accessing additional donor information. For example, brief answers about the donor's personality, interests, and aptitudes are available free of charge through the California Cryobank and are considered a "short profile." Through the Fairfax Cryobank, a short medical history is offered free of charge on the donor and his family members (his parents, siblings, offspring, maternal and paternal grandparents, aunts, and uncles). This additional information can be accessed on the Internet, and we recommend that you use this service.

3. The third tier of accessing information involves purchasing detailed multi-generational medical histories on the donors that you are seriously considering. You will note that there is a fee for this information. Personality profiles, photo-matching services, genetics counseling, and audiotapes are examples of additional information that may be available for purchase.

4. The final tier involves making the call to select your donor by purchasing his semen samples. They do not "hold" semen samples. Thus, you must purchase the quantity of vials of the donor's semen that you desire (assuming that quantity is available) in order to be certain that he will be available when you are ready to begin the inseminations. It is wise to have 3-4 candidates ranked from 1-4, in the event that your #1 candidate is not available at the time of purchase. Be prepared for that possibility, because it occurs regularly.

Given that finding the perfect donor candidate is unlikely, it is important to assess and prioritize, *before you begin screening the donors from the catalog, what characteristics are most important to you (and your partner, if applicable)*. For some, physical characteristics are essential (race, eye color, hair color, etc.). For some, medical history supersedes all else. For yet others, personality may be most important. The key is to enjoy the selection process, but also to be methodical about how you select a donor and why.

And it is important not to "put all of your eggs in one basket"—literally! Donor availability and *un*availability can be a major stressor if you invest all of your energies in one candidate and he is sold out when you make that crucial call. Therefore, reduce that stress by balancing your emotions and investment, and select several candidates that meet your standards and criteria.

OUR STORY

We learned the hard way (which, incidentally, makes us feel qualified to write this book!). Over the course of our donor insemination experience, we chose to work with both unknown donors and a known donor.

Our first choice was (and still is) working with an unknown donor through a cryobank, mainly to protect our legal and parental rights. Once we made the decision to use an unknown donor, we began checking into cryobanks. Our first doctor instructed us to go through the California Cryobank, as that was the bank that their practice worked with. Our doctor filled out the necessary authorization forms for the cryobank, while we filled out and mailed our portions in order to establish an account. During our first cycle, we naively looked at the catalogs, selected our top 5-10 candidates, and then, before making our final selection, purchased their medical histories so that we could choose the healthiest of the donors under consideration. At first we found ourselves focused on choosing a donor with similar visible characteristics to Lacy (blond hair and blue eyes) in hopes the child might prove a mix of the two of us. However, this proved almost impossible as either very few blond and blue-eyed donors were available (due to their popularity) or, oddly enough, many of them had medical histories that caused concern. We *assumed* that the donors and their immediate family members would be free of major medical problems (i.e., cancers, heart problems, liver disease, etc.), given the intense screening process used by most cryobanks. However, this was not the case, and we were very surprised to see the number of donors who had serious illnesses in multiple generations of their family. Needless to say, our priority shifted from physical characteristics to medical history quickly. In any case, we eventually narrowed down our choices and made the call to order our top choice. When we called the cryobank, all the while toasting our meticulous and seemingly wise decision-making process, we were crushed when he, and our second and third choices, were unavailable! Those particular donors had either become "inactive" (no longer providing samples for their program), were unavailable, or they only had samples that were still being quarantined for later testing. At this point we turned to the Internet for faster retrieval of information, did not invest our emotions in any of the donors, and accepted that brown eyes and brown hair were honorable characteristics!

Our first purchased donor sounded adorable. We chose him first for his squeaky clean medical history and then for his height and weight ratio. We even ordered an audiotape which solidified our decision after we heard him describe his life as a schoolteacher and his aspirations to obtain his doctorate degree. He was articulate, had a sense of humor, and sounded very grounded in his view of himself and the world. What more could we ask for?! As you may ascertain . . . we were invested! And, of course, we thought we'd get pregnant the first cycle. We purchased six vials of our donor's sperm (anticipating two inseminations per month), which our first doctor stored at their office in their own tank free of charge to patients. After three months of inseminations with this donor, no pregnancy, and the donor's unavailability at the cryobank, we dismantled the audiotape, shredded the profiles, and cried a river of tears. We found ourselves mourning the loss of this donor and questioning the reality of a family. Knowing we had to get back on the horse, we chose and purchased another donor (did not order an audiotape) and began another two cycles. When these attempts did not result in pregnancy, we began to consider a known donor.

While thinking about a known donor was scary for us, we knew who we wanted it to be without question. We had been good friends for a very long time, and he is gay, so he understood and respected our desire to become parents through donor insemination. From the beginning, he was very supportive and cooperative with respect to the details of the insemination process. He discussed the arrangement with us at length, signed sperm sale and donor agreements, and followed through on many health physicals, sexually-transmitted-diseases screenings, and fertility tests. The one obstacle was the fact that he lived on the opposite coast of the United States. So we planned a two-week adventure to his area of the country during the "optimal" window of the menstrual cycle. In between sightseeing and rock climbing we all worked together in performing several nonmedical IVI inseminations. Boy, what an exhausting process! We felt so positive about the pregnancy given the abundance of fresh sperm available on a moment's notice during *every* desired day of the cycle. When we did not achieve pregnancy this time we were devastated. It was at this point that we became crazed information seekers and discovered several important facts that doctors had never told us about the insemination procedure and getting pregnant in general (most of which are covered in other areas of this book). An additional example of vital DI trivia is the importance of *not* washing the insemination utensils in soap because the soap (or soap residue) can kill live sperm in subsequent inseminations. Rather, either use sterile utensils each time, or rinse them with only hot water. These are the little details that can have a huge impact on women's conceiving through DI.

Due to the financial and geographical constraints associated with using this known donor, we were unable to inseminate during consecutive cycles. In our minds we had planned two trips a year to visit him, planning unknown donor inseminations during the months in between. However, we did not need to visit him again as we finally achieved pregnancy shortly after our first visit with him. All in all, we found the known donor experience to be very positive, giving the majority of the credit to our known donor, who is a wonderful man. We found open and honest communication, prearranged boundaries, and a sense of humor to be the most important contributing factors to our positive view of the experience.

The month we returned from the West Coast, although devastated and exhausted, we decided to begin the process of doctor-assisted IUI from scratch. We found another medical practice closer to home after a number of frantic phone calls to every practice in the county. This practice led us to the Fairfax Cryobank in Fairfax, Virginia. We made the switch and ordered an informational packet about their services, which included a wonderful videotape about how their donors are screened and selected, and about the cryobank itself. While they did not offer some of the information we enjoyed through the California Cryobank (i.e., the short profile that was filled out in the donor's own handwriting, etc.), they offered something that we deemed even better. They updated their donor catalog *daily* on the Internet, so that we could log on and see immediately which donors had what type of sperm available that day. That was an incredible resource of information, and a great stress reducer for us, given our previously described experience with donor unavailability with the California Cryobank. And, even more importantly, they provided very brief medical histories of the donors and their families on the Internet, which could be accessed free of charge. Because medical history was our number-one criteria, this was the best cryobank service for us. Therefore, selecting our donor that resulted in our son's conception from the Fairfax Cryobank was much easier than our experience with the California Cryobank, and not nearly as stressful. In addition, since our son was born, the Fairfax Cryobank has made efforts to provide additional information on their donors, including short donor answers to interesting questions (available on the Internet) and donor audiotapes.

All in all, since we experienced IVI, ICI, and IUI, and worked with unknown donors and a known donor, we feel that we are quite qualified to assess what worked best for us throughout the process. We definitely feel IUI was the most effective insemination method, and we really enjoyed the staff at the Fairfax Cryobank and the services that they offer to their customers. Their offering brief medical histories *online free of charge* is a critical reason for our continued commitment to their organization.

Our personal, humble opinion about the two cryobanks we worked with is that, overall, the Fairfax Cryobank appears to focus more acutely on the medical backgrounds of their donors while the California Cryobank focuses more intently on the aesthetic presentation of their donors (personality, aptitudes, etc.). It is clear that both cryobanks screen their donors for a variety of reasons, and both have many wonderful services and candidates to choose from. We simply enjoyed the ability to screen and select donors based on their brief medical backgrounds provided free of charge online from the Fairfax Cryobank. Both cryobanks have a lot to offer women who desire to become parents, and each cryobank will meet different people's needs. The most significant point is that there are several options from which to choose if you are going the unknown donor route, and the ability to make choices from different options diminishes some of the stress involved in this emotional process.

Chapter Six

Choosing a Doctor

For women who anticipate pursuing IUI, or doctor-assisted ICI, selecting your doctor becomes a very important part of the DI process. In the age of Health Maintenance Organizations (HMOs) and the subsequent burden on physicians to see more patients in less time, we felt the quality of our contacts with our physicians was diminished. Patients sometimes experience the "don't ask, don't tell" treatment from their doctors, in the sense that if patients do not advocate for themselves with respect to health questions and concerns, doctors do not always take the time to thoroughly explain or investigate pertinent medical information that would help to educate and treat their patients. Given the inherent stress involved in DI, it is clear that the physician you choose to work with has a high probability of influencing your experience of stress related to this process. There are qualities to look for when choosing your family facilitator, and that is what we will discuss in this chapter.

One of the most essential factors in selecting a health practitioner is gaining an understanding of his/her commitment to DI *as a specialty*. Claiming to be a specialist in a specific area generally means that the professional has received specific training in that particular area and that they remain current with the latest research and information on that area of practice. Some doctors list DI as a specialty, but, in actuality, they know little about the evolving technological advances of the process. Some practices have one doctor in the group who has performed DI and is knowledgeable about the process, while less trained and less knowledgeable practitioners actually perform the procedure. With the emotional and financial investment that DI requires, it is very important that you find a competent physician who not only understands the process, but also remains committed to continued education in this area of practice. Your best option is to be an educated consumer. Research and understand exactly what services, skills, and "bedside manner" you are paying for. If you live in an area where there aren't many options in terms of doctors who perform DI, it is still important for you to research and assess the competencies and limitations of all the doctors with whom you anticipate working. If you do in fact identify limitations, then you will need to either: (1) choose a different practitioner, (2) assert and discuss your concerns about those limitations with that practitioner, or (3) be prepared to accept those limitations and find ways in which you are able to compensate (if possible) for his/her limitations (i.e., doing your own DI research, performing inseminations at home, etc.). Be smart, and be very selective if you can.

Second, it is important to assess the office staff. Insensitive staff who don't understand the process of DI can also raise stress levels. Ascertain in the months *before* you begin trying to conceive the level of empathy, knowledge, and basic communication skills of the receptionists, nurses, and nurse practitioners. You can do this via phone contacts and "drop by" visits. Assess who is receptive to DI patients, and who is not. If you have positive contacts with one staff member, see if you can work with them each time you need an appointment or a question answered. Assess the positive staff qualities, as well as their limitations. These issues become important on several occasions. First, the physician's assistants and other members of the office staff frequently are the ones coordinating your entire insemination. Therefore, they should demonstrate an awareness of the time constraints or urgency inherent in the process. In addition, they are often the ones who thaw or prepare your semen specimen. It is critical to have someone who understands the limitations of sperm (and thawing procedures) when you have so much invested in each precious sample. It is also important to have an understanding of the organization of your doctor's office in situations such as when you test positive to ovulate on a Friday and require a weekend insemination. Or when you must call and speak to a nurse regarding a dubious ovulation predictor test result. These members of the office staff can fuel the stressful fire or extinguish a raging flame. In the end, the doctor often only sees you for the actual procedure, while the nurses and other office staff are the front line that intercepts your phone calls and answers questions. You want to feel confident in them! Thus, make an educated choice about whether this practice as a whole can meet your family planning needs. If they cannot meet your needs entirely, consider whether you are willing to employ them based on a fraction of your needs. And if so, be clear about what that fraction is, so that you can get your outstanding needs met elsewhere. These proactive efforts can empower lesbian women, and prevent us from feeling victimized in a process that often seems so beyond our control.

OUR STORY

We cannot begin to outline all of our negative experiences with medical staff since we first began this process. But, what keeps our perception of our experience positive is the success we've had in learning how to circumvent some of these problems by educating ourselves and reducing our dependence on the medical staff for their (lack of) knowledge. Ultimately, we have learned to take charge of the process as much as possible. Despite the many problems we have had with the doctors and their staff, we still conceived our beautiful sons. And so, we will share just a few of our disheartening experiences with these doctors, hoping that they might teach you what to look out for in your quest to find a qualified, competent DI physician.

There are three situations that probably are the most poignant. The first involved several appointments for insemination in which the physician's assistants thawed our donor's sperm upon my arrival at the office. That is a normal procedure. What was problematic was that the practitioner performing the inseminations was so chatty with her other patients (oblivious to the time frame of DI and thawed sperm) that I would often sit there and watch the sperm in the syringe on the counter for an hour or more, waiting for the practitioner to arrive to perform the insemination. It was not simply an issue of being left there to wait for such an extended period of time, but more importantly, the thawed sperm generally only live and are capable of fertilizing an egg for *up to* an hour post thaw! So, many times, I questioned whether my body was receiving dead or dying sperm. This certainly did not reduce my anxiety, which in turn did not help my chances of conception.

On another occasion, one of the practitioners performing the insemination asked me what to do. Obviously, this was not a good indication that she knew what she was doing. Then, after she inserted the ICI sample and removed the speculum, half the sample came out with the speculum and ended up on the exam table. All that kept running through my mind was the intense coordinating, planning, and running around required to get me to that appointment, on the right day, at the right time, only to have an expensive sample half-wasted on the exam table. When the semen came out, I communicated to her that that was not supposed to happen. She then asked, "Boy, how expensive is a vial like that?" She proceeded to ask one of the other doctors whether sperm is supposed to fall out so quickly with the speculum, and the doctor she asked replied, "When heterosexuals have intercourse, the same thing happens." Neither practitioner had any understanding of the limitations of the DI process and frozen semen itself, the value (emotional and financial) of every drop of that sperm sample, or the clear signs of my anguish and distress at what had just occurred. No apologies were ever made, and no attempts to change the way they conducted business were ever initiated.

Finally, we inevitably encountered problems with doctors during the months when weekend inseminations were required. Some on-call doctors simply refused to do the procedure on the weekend. We never knew whether this was due to their hectic clinical or personal golf game schedule. Regardless, it is important to clarify this issue before agreeing to use a particular practice. Our frustrations were eventually rewarded when this specific practice disbanded, we assume due to patient dissatisfaction.

We cite these examples of doctor insensitivity not to scare you, but to educate you in differentiating between what is a small limitation of a doctor's practice, and what is a huge medical and ethical violation of a patient's rights. Living in an area where we felt our DI physician options were very limited, we felt as though we had to tolerate the way we were being treated in order to have a chance at getting pregnant. After feeling completely abused and victimized by this practice, Lacy "cold-called" ob-gyn offices in our area, inquiring as to whether they performed DI. When one office returned our call and reported that they did do DI, we set up a consult with a doctor. The doctor that I initially had that consult with ended up performing my insemination that conceived our firstborn son, and she ultimately ended up being the doctor on-call when we delivered! It is worth the time and energy to research your family facilitator before you begin this process. Lesbian women should not have to endure insensitive acts like the ones we described. Learn from us, and get to know what your doctor's office is really all about. Make an informed choice.

Chapter Seven

Stories from Our Sisters

Going through donor insemination for thirteen months (the first time around) was very lonely at times, as we were geographically distant from most of our family and friends. However, we did have friends around the country who were simultaneously going through the DI process, and with whom we shared a great deal. We shared our feelings, fears, and frustrations about DI. We offered words of encouragement to one another and shared our knowledge with one another . . . in the hopes that some morsel of information might help one of us actualize our dream of having a family. We want to offer a similar resource to you, to validate your struggles, stresses, and experiences.

In this chapter, we will present the stories of four couples who underwent DI or who were inseminating at the time this book was written. Sadly, we were unable to locate and interview any single lesbians about their DI experiences. Given the great diversity within our own community, we are certain that single lesbian women are pursuing DI. However, it has been *our* experience that the majority of women pursuing parenthood through DI are in coupled relationships. This may be due to the financial and emotional demands of DI and the awesome long-term responsibility of providing for and parenting the children we conceive. Committed partnerships may provide the necessary security and support that are essential in this journey. In light of the additional or special challenges single lesbian women may face, we want to take a moment and validate, support, and celebrate the single lesbian women in the world today who are taking charge of their reproductive health and defining and creating their own sense of family. Kudos to you all! We hope the following couples' stories will validate both single lesbians' and committed couples' DI experiences and this chosen path to parenthood.

COUPLE 1

Margie and Maria are 36 and 32 years old, respectively. They are a committed couple and have been together for four years. At the time of our research, they both worked full time in the fields of accounting and computer consulting. They made the decision to create their family through DI after having been together one year.

This couple tried to conceive through ICI for 6 menstrual cycles (trying both at home and with the assistance of a doctor) without success. The number-one factor that led them to cease ICI and try alternative methods was their frustration with their lack of success. Upon ceasing ICI, they pursued IUI with a fertility clinic. Simultaneously, Maria (the childbearing mother-to-be) took the fertility medication Clomid. In the third cycle with IUI and Clomid, they conceived their baby! Thus, it took them nine menstrual cycles with DI to achieve pregnancy. Each monthly cycle, Maria underwent two inseminations one to two days apart.

In addition to their Clomid and IUI efforts, Maria also had sonograms performed a couple of days prior to insemination so that her health practitioner could verify if a follicle was ready for ovulation. The average cost per insemination with these measures under their physician's care was between $600-$1,200. They received partial coverage through Maria's health insurance for these fees.

Margie and Maria chose to purchase frozen sperm from the California Cryobank for their inseminations. They decided that they felt most comfortable with an unknown donor. They "feared using a known donor because of parental rights [issues]."

To predict Maria's ovulation, they monitored her basal body temperature, cervical mucus, and ovulation predictor test results. They found the ovulation predictor kit to be their most reliable method, while her temperatures and cervical mucus were difficult to read or interpret. They stated that her temperature readings were "all over the map . . . [and that it] was difficult to see a pattern."

Maria and Margie felt that dealing with their health insurance issues, the stressful ups and downs of the DI process, and the insensitive clinic staff were the three most *emotionally challenging factors* in the overall process. They felt that the fertility clinic staff members were "very insensitive and not knowledgeable. The doctors were good but we frequently had to deal with the staff." Their most *helpful* ingredient in achieving conception was "patience. It can take awhile, and stressing out doesn't help." This couple did consider ceasing their attempts to conceive during the months without success, and planned to research adoption after twelve DI cycles. In preparation to begin DI, they read literature on the process (e.g., *The Lesbian Parenting Book*), they had a fertility consult with their doctor, and Maria began taking a prenatal vitamin. They shared their plans to have a baby with close friends and family. Both felt supported by family and friends for the most part and did not feel judged for creating their family through DI.

Margie and Maria hope to have a second child at some point through DI. They plan to start the next round with IUI and Clomid.

COUPLE 2

Linda and Juli are 32 and 39 years old, respectively. They are a committed couple and have been together for 10 years. They both worked full time in the fields of social work and exercise physiology when they began the insemination process. They made the decision to have a family within the first year of meeting each other and began trying to conceive after five years together.

This couple tried to conceive through ICI for approximately 2.5 years, without success. They tried ICI at home, and also with the aid of their physician. They inseminated only once per month, and their health insurance covered the cost of the inseminations (but not the cost of the sperm). The most significant factors that led to the cessation of attempts were their frustration with their lack of success, and, ultimately, "emotional burnout." When they stopped inseminating, they chose to adopt a baby from China. Within approximately eighteen months of deciding to adopt, they met their daughter in China and brought her home.

When trying DI, Linda and Juli chose to purchase frozen sperm from the California Cryobank. They felt much more comfortable with using an unknown donor. They provided a realistic description of their experiences with unknown donor selection:

> [Initially,] we were very selective, trying to partially match the donor to the non-childbearing partner. As cycles came and went and we needed new donors we became less selective, paying the most attention to medical and mental health issues rather than matching traits, etc.

To predict Juli's (the childbearing-mom-to-be) ovulation, they tried to track her basal body temperature, and they also used ovulation predictor tests. The basal body temperature readings "never were accurate"; her temperature charts never demonstrated the characteristic changes when she ovulated. They reported feeling that the ovulation predictor tests were their most reliable method of prediction; however, even the tests created issues of unreliability due to the degree of color change that is subjective and difficult to interpret.

Linda and Juli felt the stressful ups and downs and the waiting time for results were the most *emotionally challenging factors* for them in this process. They "felt helpless in easing the pain of disappointment" for each other. In preparation for DI in the beginning, they read literature about the process, had a fertility consult with a doctor, Juli started a prenatal vitamin, and they talked with staff at their cryobank. Juli had a fertility workup done after 6 failed attempts, including testing to see if she had any blockages or endometriosis. They shared their plans for DI with Linda's family and friends, and with one member of Juli's nuclear family. They felt that "everyone was excited for us, and had lots of questions since it was new to everyone. It was fun." They did not feel judged for creating their family through DI. "[Their] marriage was considered like any other, so wanting a family was expected."

After adopting their beautiful daughter from China, they made the decision for Juli to try again using IUI and Clomid. After two cycles and no pregnancy, they are planning to begin the adoption process again for a sibling for their daughter. The cost of their intracervical insemination procedure was $60 per insemination, and the cost of IUI (with a sonogram to test for follicle) was $200 per insemination.

Juli and Linda feel that their experiences throughout both the DI and adoption processes have "brought to light some personal vulnerabilities [they] weren't aware of." The fertility medication appears to have caused mood swings in Juli, which tested both of their abilities to be patient and tolerant. They reported that taking these paths toward parenthood has made them "stronger [people] and stronger as a couple."

COUPLE 3

Mary and Aimee are 32 and 35, respectively. They are a committed couple and have been together for nine years. At the time of our research, they both worked full time in the fields of occupational therapy and nursing. While they have been in a relationship for nine years, they made the decision to create their family through DI after having been together one year.

This couple tried to conceive through IUI for 10 menstrual cycles without success. Each monthly cycle, the childbearing-mom-to-be underwent two inseminations, twenty-four hours apart. In the eighth month, she began to take Clomid. The number-one factor that led them to cease IUI and try alternative methods was frustration with their lack of success. Upon ceasing IUI, they pursued more involved reproductive methods.

They initially worked with a physician who performed the IUI and then began inseminating at home, as Aimee is a nurse by training. The average cost for two intrauterine inseminations per month performed by their physician was $1,000 including sperm. These costs were not covered through insurance.

Mary and Aimee chose to purchase frozen sperm from the New England Cryogenic Bank for their inseminations. They decided that they felt most comfortable with an unknown donor because they "felt that legally, [it] was the easiest way to handle" the situation.

To predict the childbearing partner's ovulation, they monitored her ovulation predictor test results only. They found the ovulation predictor kit to be their most reliable method.

Mary and Aimee felt that dealing with doctor insensitivity, financial costs, fertility problems, health insurance issues, the stressful ups and downs, and the waiting involved in the DI process to be the most *emotionally challenging factors* in the overall process. Despite their lack of conception at the time this book was written, this couple has not considered ceasing their attempts to conceive.

In preparation to begin DI, they had a fertility consult with their doctor, and the childbearing partner began taking a prenatal vitamin and also had a fertility workup done. They shared their plans to have a baby with close friends and family. Both felt supported by siblings and friends, but experienced less support from their parents. They reported that at times they felt judged for deciding to create their family in this manner. "People have expressed concern about two women raising children as opposed to [a] man [and] woman raising child[ren]."

Mary and Aimee described general frustration with the entire DI process, and specifically with the lack of physicians' procedural knowledge. When asked how DI has affected their relationship, they responded with the following:

I think we both feel that it has brought us closer together. I know others have separated because of the longevity of the whole process and the emotional turmoil, but for Aimee and I, I think that it has solidified our relationship even more. I really didn't think that was possible, as we have always found support in each other through difficult times, but we both really feel directed towards having a family and will go to all extents to complete this process, [including] adoption. . . . I know for myself personally, that it has been very difficult in that I wonder if something is wrong with me, but Aimee has been very supportive, and we continue on. I don't think I could do it without her, especially since it has taken us so long.

COUPLE 4

Carrie and Paula, ages 38 and 36, respectively, are a committed couple. They have been together for five years. They both work full time; one is a CPA and the other a physician. They made the decision to have a baby through DI after being together eighteen months, but began trying to conceive after four years together.

This couple tried and successfully conceived their baby through ICI. Paula, the childbearing partner, got pregnant in the second menstrual cycle in which they inseminated. They purchased frozen sperm from the Fairfax Cryobank and chose an unknown donor for the "legal 'safety' issues regarding paternal rights." Although they used ICI, their physician performed the insemination because it is illegal in their state to do home inseminations. Their health insurance covered the cost of one insemination a month.

In order to predict ovulation, they used only one method: the ovulation predictor test kit. They felt that the most *emotionally challenging factor* in the DI process for them was making the decision to use a sperm bank, "due to fears about the process and the lack of true knowledge about the donor." However, after weighing all of their options, they decided that selecting an unknown donor through a cryobank was the safest option for them. They determined that the sperm banks appeared ethical about their screening processes, and they liked their donor's profile.

Paula and Carrie thought that the most *helpful* ingredient in their (rather speedy) conception success was Paula's "very regular" menstrual cycles and her apparent "fertility." Before they began the inseminations, they prepared themselves by reading DI literature, having a fertility consult with a doctor, taking a prenatal vitamin, and having a fertility workup done with their doctor.

They did not share their plans for DI with anyone until after inseminating and conceiving. Once they disclosed their pregnancy news, they experienced support from family and friends. There was only one issue with a family member viewing their DI decision as a "pregnancy out of wedlock." However, they report that after further communication, the issue was resolved.

Paula and Carrie commented on their feelings about DI in general. They captured our feelings perfectly in the following response:

> [it is the best] option available in a world where the ideal would be for the two of [them] to be able to conceive jointly. Obviously, biologically that cannot happen. Using brothers or friends . . . in our opinion, is risky for legal and family reasons. [The] sperm bank represented the best opportunity for us to safely conceive and have a family.

They intend to try DI again for their second child, allowing for each partner to carry a child. For now, they are enjoying their new little miracle, their daughter. In terms of the overall impact of DI on their relationship, they had this to say:

> As good as our relationship was before we embarked on this journey, it is better and stronger now. We feel profoundly and deeply connected.

Surviving the stress and strain on a relationship from the process and at times longevity of DI is a major feat. It lends credence to the old adage, *that which does not break us makes us stronger.* We celebrate the many lesbian women who are persevering in the pursuit of their family, in spite of the obstacles or challenges along the way.

Chapter Eight

Womb Wellness

It often seems that many elements in the DI process are beyond our control. Frequently, the sperm are produced by an anonymous donor, handled by a third party, shipped and delivered via Federal Express, thawed and handled by medical staff, and inseminated by a health practitioner. The egg's ability to burst from the ovary at precisely the right moment involves a highly complex interplay between hormones and internal reproductive organs. However, we are here to tell you that there are several things women *can* do to optimize their chances of conception. This chapter is devoted to addressing these issues and to empowering women to take control of their womb's wellness. Your womb will be your child's first home . . . so it is important to take steps *before you conceive* to make his/her stay as comfortable and healthy as possible!

What we call *womb wellness*, Sussman and Levitt (1989) call Prepregnancy Medicine (p. 2). According to Sussman and Levitt, these concepts essentially refer to:

> . . . alleviating [infant] disorders whose roots lie in genetics, poor nutrition, life-style, and exposures to toxic substances. . . . (p. 2)

The focus, then, is not just maximizing a woman's health once she becomes pregnant, but rather creating an optimal pregnancy environment *before* she actually conceives. The areas that we will address in order to highlight the importance of prepregnancy medicine include: diet/nutrition, exercise, drugs and alcohol, and stress reduction.

Nutrition is a very important ingredient in a woman's overall health and her chances of a healthy conception. Lauersen and Bouchez (1991) report, "by making sure you eat enough both before and after you get pregnant, [you] can increase your chances for not only a fast conception, but a healthy baby!" (p. 161). The old adage *you are what you eat* is very applicable to women's overall fertility. Lauersen and Bouchez describe the results of several National Network to Prevent Birth Defects studies, in which nutritious meal plans were found to help women fight the fertility-depleting effects of toxins found in drugs, alcohol, cigarette smoke, and air pollution (p. 161). The authors proceed to report that further studies have indicated that nutritionally balanced diets (including necessary daily quantities of vitamins and minerals) can reduce a woman's risk of problems when she is pregnant. Nutrition can therefore potentially affect women's experience of labor, hypertension, gestational diabetes, and excessive bleeding (Lauersen & Bouchez, 1991, p. 161).

In addition to eating the right foods in the proper quantities, avoiding certain foods during the preconception period may also assist your fertility. It is recommended by many doctors and sources of fertility information that women planning to conceive avoid artificial sweeteners, soda pop, fruit drinks that are high in sugar, candy, rare red meat, hot dogs (and other processed meats), and products containing caffeine. Each of these foods, for different reasons, has the ability to interfere with your reproductive health and your chances of conception. For more information on the effects of nutrition on women's fertility, or for recommended meal plans, check out the work of Eisenberg, Murkoff, and Hathaway (1991), Lauersen and Bouchez (1991), and/or Sussman and Levitt (1989).

Exercise is another factor within our control. Overall, the literature suggests that being in good physical condition prior to conception can assist your having a healthier pregnancy. However, too much of any one thing can sometimes be counterproductive. *Everything in moderation.* Lauersen and Bouchez (1991) report that:

. . . . some strenuous activities work against female fertility. They can cause a variety of negative effects, from menstrual irregularities to outright infertility, for nearly all women of childbearing age. (p. 152)

The strenuous activities they are referring to include marathon or triathlon training, excessive jogging, and intense high-energy aerobics on a regular basis. They state that engaging in these activities regularly can have an impact on your reproductive health by interfering with egg production and ovulation. They report that research on exercise has demonstrated that

requiring you to push your body too hard for too long a period of time may inhibit the functioning of your hypothalamus gland, and in the process upset the function of timing of all reproductive hormones necessary for conception. (p. 153)

While there are risks for the extreme forms of exercise, a balanced exercise routine can aid your fertility. Mild, aerobic activities that contribute to your overall conditioning are recommended. These activities include swimming, walking, bicycling, and stretching (Lauersen & Bouchez, 1991, p. 155). These types of milder exercises can help keep you fit, while not interfering with the delicate hormonal balance in your body.

In addition to nutrition and exercise, drugs and alcohol are important risk factors that can be controlled. Common sense tells us that chemicals found in street drugs or alcohol are not conducive to a healthy womb and pregnancy, and should be strictly prohibited. Over-the-counter drugs or prescription medications should be discussed with your doctor. When the benefits of modern medicine for mothers at risk for certain medical problems greatly outweigh the risk to an anticipated baby, your physician can discuss these issues with you and help you to make a decision in the best interest of the family. However, overall, where medications (prescription or otherwise), alcohol, and other recreational drugs are concerned, it is best to abstain throughout the preconception period as well as throughout pregnancy.

Last, but certainly not least, is the importance of reducing your stress. Stress affects our body's balance and functioning power. It can affect our immune system, energy levels, mental health, and fertility. While some degree of stress is inherent in the DI process, there are ways to minimize or eradicate the stress from our environment. Lauersen and Bouchez (1991) claim that because "[stress] is capable of causing everything from brief menstrual upset to complete, and sometimes permanent, cycle shutdown," women must work to identify the causes of their stress and then seek to remove the source of stress from their lives (p. 157). They suggest that to do this, women should assess their lives and identify the smaller, more manageable stressors that the major ones comprise. Women can often address, contain, and/or eliminate these smaller stressors in order to create a more relaxed atmosphere. In addition to working to "not sweat the small stuff," these authors recommend taking additional mental health time for one's self. Whenever possible, reduce some of the daily stress by setting aside time for a hot, relaxing bath, a massage, napping, journaling, or reading a good book.

Another important Lauersen and Bouchez concept is assessing whether any "hidden stress" exists in your life. They make the point that tension, depression, and hectic schedules have become a part of daily living, and often women do not attend to how much stress is actually alive and at work in their lives. They recommend utilizing your menstrual cycle as a gauge of your hidden stress. Despite how you might feel, irregular menstrual cycles and other tension-related menstrual issues like cramps and backaches could be a sign of some form of stress-related fertility problem. If you detect any irregularities, they recommend having a consult with your doctor for further evaluation and treatment planning (p. 158).

OUR STORY

While nutrition is a very important preconception factor, we only made a few changes to my daily diet. Innately, it seems, I am a pretty "healthy" eater; my diet is essentially free from caffeine (no soda, no chocolate, no coffee), diet beverages and foods containing aspartame, and other nutritional and gestational hazards. Thus, avoiding foods that potentially affect fertility was not an issue for me.

However, two changes we did make in terms of my diet included changing my vitamin and increasing my protein intake. I started taking a prenatal vitamin after our preconception planning consult with the doctor and ceased all other vitamin supplements. In addition, I altered my fairly vegetarian diet by adding proteins such as tuna fish, egg salad, cottage cheese, yogurt, and chicken. Adding these foods was a little bit of a challenge because I have been known to be a "picky" eater and often remain within my comfort zone of favorite foods. I committed to myself and Lacy that, for fertility's sake, I would eat more frequently and substantially to keep my weight on track and to provide my body, the baby vessel, with the nurturance that conception and pregnancy would require. Interestingly, once I became pregnant, not only did my appetite soar to levels previously unimaginable, but I actually enjoyed new tastes, spices, and textures! Thus, altering my diet before conception actually facilitated the transition into the nutritional demands of pregnancy!

In addition to nutrition, we made efforts to moderate my exercise routines. Having been active athletes in college, we had to tone down our choice of athletic endeavors from lacrosse and tennis to mild aerobic activities and walking. Feeling fit prior to conception allowed us to enjoy a complication-free pregnancy and delivery.

Drugs–over-the-counter, prescription, and otherwise–as well as alcohol were not an issue for this "Sandra Dee." When I had colds or mild headaches, I chose not to seek out over-the-counter medicines, just to be on the safe side. Instead, I would choose warm baths, hot compresses, and salt water gargling to relieve the symptomatology.

Stress was our biggest enemy in this process, and stress reduction was a difficult goal to attain. It took some time and extra effort to learn how to change the things we could and accept the things we couldn't. We engaged in extensive "partner communication therapy," as we like to call it, in which we each shared our frustrations and anticipations for that cycle. Talking and sharing our anxieties provided relief most of the time. Talking it out definitely helped to detoxify the stress that so persistently wanted to take hold of our mental and physical health. We also found different types of healthy distractions in our lives during peak stress periods, in an effort to balance our energy input and output regarding the DI process. We really relied on the strength of our partnership to alleviate much of the stress, stepping up to support each other and finding ways to handle it together.

Researching the process (in moderation) helped to reduce our stress levels, as much of our stress seemed to be directly linked to feeling ignorant about DI. Reading fertility literature sometimes empowered us, subsequently dissipating the stress. This was not true all of the time, because occasionally Lacy tried to avoid anxiety by *not* reading or talking out her feelings. This difference in our styles of handling anxiety promoted conflict. Ultimately, we learned to negotiate a balance between information-seeking and information obsession. We also learned to respect the different ways we each cope with stress in our lives.

Thus, the greatest stress reducer, above all else, was having each other and feeling the true meaning of partnership.

Chapter Nine

Who Will Carry?

It is obvious that with the DI process, no woman can ever claim "Whoops! I accidentally got pregnant!" We know that DI requires extensive forethought, planning, decision making, communicating, and coordinating. And so, for lesbian couples, deciding who will physically carry the baby demands equal attention, in terms of its emotional and physical considerations. While this chapter is devoted to addressing this important decision for couples, single lesbians can benefit from answering some of the questions posed in the "decision trees" as well. All of the issues are presented in an effort to further clarify each woman's role in, readiness for, and commitment to the DI process.

In talking with other couples, we found that more often than not the choice to carry ends up being a fairly easy one. It seems that most often one partner is the likely choice given level of desire, age, fitness, etc. The desire to be pregnant and give birth is usually stronger in one partner, and it is this partner who carries, or at least tries first! However, this is not always the case. When both partners have an equal emotional and physical desire to carry a baby, some important factors must be considered when deciding who will conceive. We believe level of desire and commitment to carry a child should be first and foremost when making such an important decision. The road ahead promises to be a long one and the carrier needs to be prepared for dietary restrictions, physical changes to the body, invasive medical procedures, possibly physical discomfort and pain, and periods of emotional instability. It is a monumental commitment not only to the baby, but also to the spouse and to one's self.

In addition to the psychological component of the decision, there are very real and practical factors that must be considered when choosing who will carry. These include issues of fertility and family health history. The following are some questions to prepare you and your partner to assess fertility. We will apply concepts described previously in the book.

1. Is the length of your menstrual cycle consistent across months? Do you have "routine cycles"?
2. Are you ovulating? If so, are you ovulating in a predictable fashion each month (confirmed by tracking results from BBT, CM, the Os, and OPKs)?
3. Has your menstrual cycle been problematic over the years, causing cramps, unusual flow, etc.?
4. Have any other women in your family had fertility problems? Have they had any other reproductive disorders such as miscarriages or endometriosis?
5. Is your work environment safe and relatively toxin-free? (Do you work with chemicals, lift heavy equipment, or experience high levels of work-related stress?)
6. Is your body weight within preconception guidelines?
7. Is your age a fertility factor, or a factor for potential pregnancy complications or birth defects?
8. Is your lifestyle conducive to protecting the unborn? (Do you eat nutritiously, avoid alcohol and drugs, and avoid risky behaviors?)

These questions are designed to encourage each partner to think about her capacity to conceive, nurture the pregnancy, and eventually give birth to a healthy baby.

In addition to evaluating fertility issues en route to choosing a carrier, it is important to explore each partner's family health history. Since lesbian couples do have the choice of two women instead of one, we believe it is important to consider avoiding the possibility of major familial health problems. Clearly, if one of you has battled cancer or another long-term, possibly fatal illness, it may be wise to leave the childbearing to the other partner. This is not only to avoid passing on the propensity for the illness to the child but also to also relieve the physical and emotional burden which could exacerbate any illness. We also found it important to interview family members and gain a working knowledge of the existing physical and mental health problems in not only the immediate family but also a couple of generations back (including parents, siblings, aunts, uncles, cousins, grandparents, etc.). This is all information you will be gathering about the donor, so why not be thorough and explore your histories, not only to make a smart decision about who will carry, but also to gain a broader picture of that future child as well?

Not only are desire, fertility, and family health histories crucial to this important decision, but the practical aspects of pregnancy must be considered as well. These often consist of concerns that most couples are unaware of or do not consider at all, such as health insurance issues, maternity leave coverage, safety and job protection, overall health, and income. The following questions are designed to stimulate your mind to think about specific, practical issues that might otherwise have been left out of the decision-making process:

1. Do you both have health insurance? Which plan has better maternity coverage? Or are they both equal?
2. What are your maternity leave benefits through employment? Which partner has a better package?
3. Who can be home part time or full time after the baby is delivered if that is an option or priority?
4. Of the two partners, who thinks that they could feel and be safe when pregnant at work? Safe in terms of building hazards, toxic material exposure, high-stress environments, and freedom from hate crimes/violence?
5. Do you each feel that your job, your position and status at work, will be protected while on leave if you plan to return to the workforce full time after delivery and recovery?

6. Do you each feel physically capable of handling the demands of pregnancy on your body? Are there any health issues that could complicate the pregnancy for either one of you?
7. If the partner chosen to carry the child is the major breadwinner in the family, can you afford loss of pay or reduced pay for the time in which she might have unpaid maternity leave?

Answers to these questions may help refine the issue of who will carry. While most of them are easy to answer, they are often forgotten or avoided due to their practicality in an otherwise very emotional decision.

Ideally, the evaluation of all these major aspects of each partner's life will lead to an obvious conclusion about who will carry the child. If the issue continues to remain undecided, and all factors appear equal for each person, then perhaps the agreement will be for both to carry at some point in the relationship. In the end, we feel the decision should be in the best interest of the child; therefore, all of the aforementioned factors, including fertility issues, age, overall health, and level of desire, should be compared and contrasted thoroughly and selflessly.

OUR STORY

In our case, the decision to carry was natural and obvious. I had always had a strong desire to be pregnant, and Lacy had not. While she very much wanted to be a parent, she did not necessarily desire to endure all the demands of pregnancy and delivery. In addition, she has a longstanding history of irregular and painful menstrual cycles. This, combined with her age (33), meant a lot of fertility testing, possibly medication to induce regular cycles, and medical procedures to validate ovulation. Given her lack of confidence in the medical profession, these facts alone dissipated her desire quickly! Thus, many factors seemed to lend credence to my carrying the child(ren).

Another major consideration was the fact that Lacy not only is the breadwinner of the family but also works as a psychologist in a prison setting. Clearly, this presented two issues: financial concerns and physical safety. We could not afford to have children in the first place if Lacy weren't bringing home a paycheck, and the risk to Lacy's physical safety in her work environment was not conducive to ensuring a stress-free pregnancy.

While all of these factors seemed to add up to a logical choice, it was not without struggle. Lacy admits her core struggle with the decision was not only her desire to pass on her own genes, but also her family's subtle pressure to "bear the Frazer fruit." Lacy held the common belief that her parents were eager for *her* to carry a child in the future because of their desire for a biological grandchild. In the end, after much communication and sharing of feelings, we eventually agreed to my carrying the first child (and ultimately the second as well). We have thoroughly discussed and agreed on ways to parent the children, to reinforce our goal of 100% parental equality and responsibility regardless of biological ties.

Chapter Ten

The Other Half:
A Nonbiological Parent's Experience of DI

While single lesbian women may choose to parent their child on their own, the role of the nonbiological parent in committed partnerships deserves special attention. I (Lacy) suppose the journey of the nonbiological parent begins with the decision to forfeit carrying the child. We described in the previous chapter our many reasons for selecting Marie as our "vessel of choice," so I will not burden you with redundancy. However, it is important to note that regardless of how easy the choice is to make, the nonbiological parent inevitably faces having to accept the ramifications of such a decision. These ramifications might include mourning the notion you may never physically carry a child, never pass on your own genetic material, and never be biologically related to your child. However, I believe these issues, once recognized and discussed, can become less important as the role of parent becomes more clearly defined and equalized with your partner.

The most prominent and important ramification that the nonbiological parent must anticipate and understand is the adoption of the role of supportive and empathetic partner. "Non-bio" parents do not have to endure uncomfortable medical evaluations and procedures, nor the stress of taking their temperature at the same time every day. They are not the ones examining cervical mucus and physically checking the diameter of the Os. They are not the ones who must prepare the body for the long, difficult task of sustaining and nourishing a human fetus for nine months. These responsibilities are numerous and often contribute to a high level of stress in both partners, with the bulk of the anxiety resting with the woman trying to get pregnant, given it is her body "under construction." And, as our medical and psychological community has taught us over the years, stress is thought to contribute to many mental and physical problems, including infertility. Thus, the role of the supportive, empathetic partner is crucial in minimizing the stress that might influence the chances of conception!

Hopefully, this supportive role starts to take shape at the beginning of any relationship, eventually becoming the foundation of the relationship, and is most useful and important during times of high stress in the relationship. Attempt at conception and eventual pregnancy is one such time! I definitely can say that it was during our "road to conception" when Marie and I experienced our most tenuous emotional time together. In general, I found myself empathizing with all she was going through; however, it remained difficult to understand the anxiety she faced on a daily basis. To make matters worse, my way of avoiding the discomfort of anxiety was to minimize the issues or avoid them altogether, which included, at times, evading discussions about preconception preparation and details. This was not helpful to Marie and often led to arguments, the perception being that I was "not invested" or "not caring enough." While it was unfortunate that we had to endure many cycles of inseminations, it was with each new cycle that we discovered new ways of coping with disappointment as well as relating with each other.

As described, the nonbiological parent faces many issues throughout the preinsemination, conception, pregnancy, and parenting stages. And it is the coping strategies employed by each individual partner that will define how the two negotiate their way to and through parenthood. Each phase of the process had its challenges for me, and I think it is important to share my experiences in hopes of preparing others for their journey. It is our *perception* of our DI experiences that differentiates the biological and nonbiological parent.

I define the preinsemination phase as the "information-gathering" stage. This was the time when we began investigating how we were going to start a family. I decided it was pretty cut and dried . . . we find a cryobank, order sperm, insert the sample, and let nature take its course. However, Marie approached things differently, ordering several books on fertility, contacting cryobanks across the country, and discussing logistical issues with the doctors. She also began to cleanse her body and prepare for pregnancy, cutting out many "toxic" foods and drinks. It felt like the more Marie read and prepared for the inseminations, the more anxious I got. I now know that this was due to the fact that, as time went by, I realized this was really going to happen and I began to question my readiness for parenthood. This question became the focus of the preinsemination stage. Was I ready to take on the responsibility of becoming a parent? This is a question that needs to be very seriously addressed long before decisions about who is going to carry the child are made. I found that as the nonbiological partner, and as a woman who did not have the intense instinct to bear a child, I had not given the decision the consideration it deserved from the beginning. And I was not being fair to Marie, having not admitted to her my fear about what lay ahead. We spent many nights getting in touch with our hopes, fears, dreams, and anxieties related to pregnancy and parenting. These issues largely included questions about familial and societal reactions to our plans, as well as our own recognition that life was going to change drastically. Were we prepared for these changes? Some examples of questions we asked ourselves included:

- How are we going to prepare our child for a world full of intolerance and judgment?
- What are some things that we can do to help minimize the obstacles our child might face as he/she grows up in a household with two mommies?
- How are we going to teach our child tolerance, patience, and the importance of unconditional love?
- How are we going to explain to the child as he/she grows older about the choices and methods we employed to start a family?

While the answers to these questions are personal and individualized, the questions themselves are largely universal and must be asked in order to ground the experience of donor insemination and its ramifications in reality for both partners. In the end, while discussing such important issues was anxiety provoking, it brought us closer together and enabled us to make sound decisions that *we* (not family and friends) felt good about.

In sum, I found there to be three important issues for me (as the non-bio parent) during the preinsemination and subsequent stages. The first is to be mindful of how my partner and I handle anxiety; the second is to make sure that I explore my feelings about the insemination process and ultimately parenthood with my partner; and third, that I make an effort to understand what she will endure en route to carrying and birthing our child.

The insemination process itself was by far the most difficult for both of us. And as the non-bio partner, it was the most grueling. This was the time when the role of supportive, empathetic partner became so important (and this is a time when single lesbian women will need to lean on their coach). As the inseminations themselves transformed from romantic, powerful experiences full of love to cold, medical procedures full of anxiety, I often transformed from an empathetic spouse to a seemingly homicidal maniac. It was virtually impossible for me to be present during the first round of physician-assisted inseminations due to my work schedule. I worked an hour west of our residence and the physician's office was 45 minutes to the east, thus requiring several hours off work in order to attend the appointments. We made the decision that Marie would conquer the appointments on her own, which soon became a nightmare. It was very difficult for me to be at work knowing she had to make a long drive to the office, face the emotionally draining incompetence of the physician and staff, and then make the long drive home . . . all the while second guessing whether or not a minute sample of sperm worth $200 was inside her or dripping onto the examining table. I began to dread the post-insemination phone call which often left me feeling sad and completely helpless as Marie sobbed on the other end of the phone, recounting how the "inseminator" and other office staff made her feel insignificant and unknowledgeable. To compound the emotional pressure inside of me was the fact that we decided not to disclose our choice to begin inseminating to my work colleagues or family members (for a variety of reasons). I was thus forced to anticipate and deal with these phone calls completely on my own and had to work hard not to let the emotions seep into my decision-making abilities at work.

Eventually, as previously discussed, Marie and I made the decision to investigate other medical practices closer to our home (something we had not done sooner because we made the assumption that the practices in our small, conservative town would not welcome a lesbian couple). We found relief in a practice a few blocks from our house. This made it more feasible for me to attend the appointments if possible and/or to feel more at ease about Marie traveling to the appointments. We still faced some office staff who were insensitive to the nuances of the procedures; however, having the office so close by seemed to minimize the trauma.

In addition to my absence at the appointments and the inevitable phone calls from a distance, we struggled a great deal with the stress of the ovulation predictor kits. On more than one occasion, Marie was forced to "read" the test with her own set of subjective eyes, as I was often at work during the hour she was required to complete the test. Because the tests relied on color shade, Marie was forced to make a determination of whether or not the test line was "the same as or darker than" the control line. It was very stressful for me at work to hear the indecisiveness regarding a test that was crucial to our successful conception. A false reading and we could have missed ovulation altogether!

As previously stated, Marie and I learned something new with every failed cycle. We felt ourselves transforming into smarter consumers, more educated patients, and a stronger team as the months went by. With every problem or stressor, we tried to devise a solution aimed at avoiding or minimizing the anxiety. For example, I began to handle the phone calls to the cryobank to purchase the samples and make shipping arrangements, as well as the calls to the physician's office to set up insemination appointments. The stress associated with battling the office staff in order to make appointments in an otherwise booked schedule or dealing with the person responsible for shipping the used tank back to the cryobank was more than Marie needed to deal with while trying to get pregnant. In addition, I made it a priority to attend all insemination appointments whenever humanly possible. This was done not only to support Marie but also to send a message to the staff that we were a united couple and committed to the process. Attending the appointments also allowed me to run interference when a disagreement in procedure arose, taking the burden off Marie.

In hindsight, I can say that open communication between the two of us was the key in mastering the obstacles of the insemination process. It was crucial for us to share our fears and anxieties, as naming them allowed us to devise solutions for conquering them. Although I was not physically going through the process, I still found a way (with Marie's help and support) to be an equal partner in this venture. And with persistence and patience we announced "we" were pregnant in April 1999!

Now, I am sure the reader realizes that I cannot stop here in my discussion of my role as the non-bio parent/partner. Pregnancy, labor, and delivery required just as much energy, empathy, and support! Pregnancy was by far the most enjoyable stage of this process. The emotional conflict (can and will we ever get pregnant?) surrounding the inseminations was over, which allowed us to return to relating to each other in a softer, more intimate way. We felt ourselves traveling down the other side of the mountain, which was hugely relieving. As the non-bio partner, I found such satisfaction and joy in helping to prepare and sustain Marie's body for a healthy pregnancy. This required me to be highly sensitive to her needs, which seemed to change on a daily basis. These included helping her walk up the steps, lifting anything over 20 lbs., cooking her healthy meals, running to the store for unexpected cravings, massaging her feet and lower back, and monitoring her physical and emotional changes. During this stage, we began discussing and making decisions about the baby's name, the nursery, and parenting issues. All of these things were very important in establishing a connection to the child and the idea of us as a family. Although I was not biologically related to or physically carrying the child, we made every effort to ensure attachment.

As with any spouse of a pregnant woman, I was a nervous wreck anticipating the labor and delivery of our child. However, this was not only due to the obvious, but also a result of worry about discrimination as a lesbian couple while at the hospital. In anticipation of possible discrimination, we made sure to discuss our situation with the nursing staff so there would be no problems with having me in the delivery room. In addition, we prepared our wills, living wills, and power of attorneys prior to the birth to ensure my ability to make any major medical decision should complications arise. Once we had these things in place we felt more secure about the entire birthing process.

It seemed as the weeks went by, giving way to the impending birth, Marie became more relaxed and serene while I became more and more anxious. I feared complications with the birth and possible poor health of the child and questioned my capabilities as a parent. I remained distracted at work and anxious at home. Finally, the contractions began and we went into the hospital. I spent the hours of Marie's labor in the bathroom with "the runs" as she slept, watched television, and discussed her lack of fear about the delivery. She was so calm! When Jack was born, I felt an indescribably amazing rush of happiness, excitement, and love instantaneously. As I helped cut the cord, I watched this little being give one small cry, then open his eyes and take in his new surroundings. The day was ours. We both began to cry and I felt the emotions of the last 21 months erupt in both of us like a volcano dormant for 100 years. This child was a miracle!

In our society today, the definition of parenthood is not limited to heterosexual couples with children. The definition encompasses a variety of different familial relationships, including lesbian mothers. Although I am not the biological mother of our children, I am their parent. I feed them, bathe them, clothe them, play with them, sleep with them, laugh with them, read to them, and love them. As a result of many important, mutual decisions along the way, Marie and I are equal parents, bearing the same amount of responsibility for their lives. Some of these decisions included bottle feeding, legal guardianship and adoption, health insurance coverage (my plan), and revising all legal documentation such as wills to include our children. While these decisions do not make them any more biologically related to me, they help ensure a sense of safety, confidence, and commitment to my role as a parent.

I have no regrets about not physically carrying either child, and I attribute this to our committment to communicate and explore the intense emotions associated with these crucial decisions *before* the onset of the insemination process.

Chapter Eleven

Parenting Today

While the majority of this book is devoted to educating readers about donor insemination and related issues, we feel this book would not be complete without a discussion on parenting our children in today's intolerant world. As a psychologist in a correctional setting, I (Lacy) am reminded daily of the significant influence environment has on the development of one's personality, behavioral motivations, and establishment of belief systems. In fact, one of my "toughest" patients, a 23-year-old, African American male serving 16 years for drug dealing, describes a life of criminal behavior rooted in survival. His views of the world are perfectly in tune with his upbringing, a childhood characterized by a lack of parental control, minimal love and nurturance, inadequate financial resources, and the need to protect at all costs. He feels bitter and angry most of his waking moments–the only emotions he is capable of expressing given that they are the only emotions he was taught as a child. He was taught at an early age that violence is the only way to solve problems and that hate will always protect you from feeling hurt. When I confront him about changing, he inevitably answers, "But this is the only way I know how to feel."

In the wake of this inmate's story, the victims of Oklahoma City, and the shootings at Columbine High School, there is a reaffirmation of the vital role that our home environment and parental attachments play in shaping who we are and who we will become. Parents can be the single most important influence on a child, because they model the behaviors absorbed by children every day. Thus, the physical and emotional environment into which a child is born will have a huge influence on who he/she becomes as

an adult. The beliefs and attitudes of the parents are formed by their pre-
ceding caregivers' views and so on, which all ultimately are influenced by
the prevailing views of society at large. Thus, the views of parents are often
adopted by their children, and this is how positive feelings and good will or
hate and discrimination are disseminated over the course of time. Parents
have the power to shape future generations.

And so, we, as prospective parents, must consider the unique challenges
of parenting children as lesbian women and as lesbian mothers. Our children not only will have lesbian parents, but also will have been conceived
through donor insemination, two inherent differences that will be a part of
their identity and their search to "fit in" among their peers and in society.
Given these facts, we must explore how we might handle people's igno-
rance, and how we will teach our children to handle such difficult personal-
ities and situations. Two key questions present themselves at this juncture.
Are we prepared to continue to self-improve, evolve, and educate ourselves to handle the changing world and worldviews around us? And are
we prepared to continue to teach and support our children, to help them to
learn, evolve, cope, manage, make decisions, respect, and interact in this
world of diversity that sometimes is comprised of intolerant human beings?

Clunis and Green (1995) describe the challenges of lesbian parenting in
their book, *The Lesbian Parenting Book: A Guide to Creating Families and
Raising Children*. They state that:

> [as] lesbian families, we challenge the very foundation upon which
> the notion of family has been based, namely heterosexuality. . . .
> Children in lesbian families, as well as the adults, have to deal with
> coming out or not, how to be and to whom. . . . (pp. 12-13)

It is unforeseeable at this point what situations and issues we and our children will face in our lifetime. However, one thing is sure: we will always
need to keep growing, exploring, communicating, and evolving to be able

to handle life's uncertainties, societal issues surrounding unconventional families, and parenting issues.

Clunis and Green make the point that while lesbian parents often lack role models, there are many advantages to being able to create our own definition of family. We are pioneers in this relatively new territory, challenging societal constraints, beliefs, and conventions. We can give our children a whole new breed of role models. Our children will absorb the positive egalitarian relationships that lesbian women share, experience the flexibility of the lesbian parents' sharing of household and parental responsibilities (as opposed to conventional heterosexual gender-assigned tasks), internalize the special strength and commitment required of single lesbian moms, and learn a way of life that is respectful of team work, equality, communication, flexibility, resiliency, and open-mindedness.

In creating a new definition of family and its structure, we have the opportunity to handle age-old parenting dilemmas with a new twist of creativity, positive energy, and effective communication skills. Some situations that arise regarding our children will be common, everyday experiences of kids their age . . . and some situations will be lesbian-specific. If we can use the skills that once helped us to surmount our own sexual-identity-forming processes and that led to the successful planning and actualization of our children, these same skills can serve us well in the parenting arena. These former self-improvement/actualization skills and insights, acquired through these challenging experiences, can translate into positive parenting skills. The following outline includes suggestions for forming new, positive family ground rules, and they are based on our own personal growth experiences. From this list, you can expand the ideas to meet your particular needs and situations.

- Create a safe environment in which all family members can be vulnerable and admit their shortcomings, failures, questions, and fears.
- Maintain a willingness to view all sides of a story (at the same time, teaching the skill of empathy for others' perceptions and actions).

- Communicate all levels of thoughts and feelings (good, bad, superficial, intense, scary, curious, indifferent, exhilarating).
- Encourage and respect appropriate emotional expression, free of gender-role stereotyping.
- Discuss and develop multiple creative solutions to challenging situations, in order to provide a sense of empowerment through options.
- Facilitate decision-making processes through teaching the power of choice and outlining the consequences of our choices.
- Teach how and when to find additional supportive resources.

As we review the previous list of options for creating a safe, structured, loving home environment, it is clear that the inmate presented at the opening of this chapter did not have such a positive childhood experience. Needs weren't met, safety was not always ensured, and unconditional love was not a mainstay in his life. Coping skills were developed in order to survive this harsh, cold environment into which he was born. And, in turn, he has mirrored to society these harsh lessons that his "caregivers" taught him.

Lesbian parents who are forced to battle societal disapproval for the very right to be true to our homosexual identity, and who face the uphill challenge of creating our families through donor insemination, demonstrate incredible character strength and resiliency through our ability to continue loving and believing in the children we will bring into this world. We have the ability to raise productive, loving, tolerant, intelligent, inquisitive children, and to shape their developing self-concept into a whole, giving, positive, authentic adult identity. Despite certain factions of society who would like to think the homosexual community does not exist, we are in fact multiplying *daily*. Although we cannot change societal views all at once, we can work to improve smaller issues in our lives which can cumulatively add up to evolutionary societal change in the long term.

As lesbian parents, we must be honest with ourselves and our children about who we are and how our children came to be. Encouraging a foundation of truthfulness is just one small way that we can teach our children important, core values. Building on the example of honesty as a value can perhaps change the lives of our children's generation by teaching them to respect courageous individuals who live truthfully and authentically, despite many bitter and judgmental people. Many issues will cross our paths in the coming years, and we have the responsibility to our kids and future generations to try to make this world a more accepting, whole, integrated place to live.

This parenthood journey is a major rite of passage for heterosexuals and homosexuals alike. And for lesbian women, it is perhaps even more significant, because "the great lesbian sperm chase" (as Clunis and Green [1995] call it) can be a very challenging pursuit that we must overcome in order to actualize our parenting dreams (p. 24). We ask you to celebrate and validate your own passage rites on this front and allow yourselves to stand in awe of the amazing feats that you are accomplishing. What an exciting time in our lives, in history, and for our community!

Chapter Twelve

Trying Again

Given the stress that accompanies DI, it is an awesome phenomenon that many lesbians persist and endure the intensity of the process until they achieve pregnancy. I remember the huge sense of joy and relief the first time my pregnancy test finally turned positive! We put away all of my BBT charts, the thermometer, and practically our DI-filled brains! The financial burden of the monthly costs of inseminations was lifted. And we sat in amazement considering the irony of DI, in which we felt *relieved* of the financial burden at conceiving our son while our heterosexual peers at this point have just begun to feel financial anxieties about the baby expenses to come. In this respect, the DI process perhaps is a good training camp for the budgeting most first-time parents encounter. In any case, we were surprised to find ourselves ready to begin undergoing inseminations for the second time when our son was just four months old.

Having known quantities, in our doctor, our cryobank, our local hospital, our attorney, my health insurance, flexible work schedules, and my overall health and fertility, was a significant factor in our desire and confidence in trying again. This, combined with a sense of always wanting to have two children, led to our making the decision to work the process again.

We tried two cycles with two back-to-back IUI inseminations, paired with taking Clomid. Both cycles failed to end in conception, and, in hindsight, we know exactly why. We decided not to rely on the OPKs initially in this second round, mainly in an attempt to reduce our stress in interpreting the test results. Instead, we counted on the predictability of the fertility medication Clomid, my BBT charts, and CM. Having had our son, we obviously suffered a clear case of feeling invincible, thinking that we were immune to the stress and limitations of DI. How quickly our egos were snapped back into the reality of DI's unpredictability!

In the third cycle, we chose to follow our own advice and employ all of the fertility tracking methods, relying heavily on the Clomid and OPKs to predict the perfect window of ovulation that is so critical to conception success. When our OPK turned positive on day 13 of my cycle, we made two morning IUI insemination appointments with our doctor, for days 14 and 15. By the morning of day 16, my temperature had risen in stairstep fashion and my Os was sealed shut. Fourteen days later, my temperature still high on my BBT chart, we were elated to see a positive pregnancy test result! In hindsight, we definitely endorse the use of multiple methods of fertility tracking when possible, especially the OPK—which has been a key ingredient in our ability to conceive our children!

The main point we want to convey in this chapter is to find what works for you, in terms of facilitating conception and addressing any feelings of frustration with the process (if applicable) before trying again. There is the potential to feel re-traumatized by the necessities of the process, the logistics as well as the emotional investment. And so, if DI the first time around was challenging emotionally for you, try to name, release, and resolve your stress before trying to conceive again. We carry our stress in our bodies, and it surfaces in ways such as illness, fatigue, depression, and fertility issues. If you work to protect and ensure your womb's wellness through a peaceful mind/body connection, you may in fact increase your chances of a smooth second conception.

Another significant issue to consider is the planning of inseminations (including ovulation tracking methods as well as the inseminations themselves) while caring for your other child(ren). We can attest to the fact that it was much easier, logistically, planning for and enduring the inseminations when we were simply dealing with our own schedules. When you have a little one, who perhaps wakes up in the middle of the night, it is important to consider who will tend to the baby in light of the constraints related to BBT monitoring. The woman being inseminated, and whose cycle is being tracked, does not want to engage in any middle-of-the-night activities that can affect her temperature readings in the morning. In addition, coordinating inseminations with the doctor's office (if applicable) presents new challenges when parents have to address the issue of childcare or bringing the child to the appointment. For lesbian couples, both partners then may need to be present for each insemination, to provide emotional support and childcare and to allow the partner being inseminated time to relax on the examining table after the insemination. For single lesbians, your DI coach or a supportive friend may need to provide daycare or meet other needs when appropriate and necessary. The issue of childcare is just something to consider when you try again, because it adds an entirely new dimension to the logistics involved in the process.

Although I can say we were disappointed at not conceiving in the first two cycles of trying DI again, we were not as emotionally depleted and anxious as we were before our first baby was conceived. There was peace in knowing that we had already established my fertility and that we were already proud parents of a beautiful baby boy. This fact alone was a magnificent source of stress reduction when we tried again.

Chapter Thirteen

The Adoption Option

Any lesbian woman or couple will want to consider the legal issues surrounding DI. For those choosing to co-parent their child with another person, the information presented in this chapter should be reviewed carefully. We understand that the mere excitement and anticipatory anxiety about succeeding in conceiving and delivering a baby may make the legal considerations regarding a nonbiological parent's relationship to the child seem light years away. But for those who are interested in gaining a broader perspective of the entire process, we feel as though we would be falling short of our responsibilities to educate women about *all* segments of DI if we did not address adoption issues. The issues of legal guardianship and co-adoption will therefore be described and discussed in this chapter.

In typical heterosexual marriages, the husband and wife are granted immediate parental rights to their offspring the minute the child is born. However, this is not the case for lesbian couples or single lesbian women seeking to involve a parenting partner. The partner who is inseminated and eventually delivers the baby is considered the biological and *only* parent of that child by the courts and anyone of legal authority. Consider the following scenario to illustrate this point. If the pregnant partner, during delivery, experiences life-threatening complications and loses consciousness, the nonbiological lesbian partner's rights (at that point) to make decisions not only about her partner but also about the medical treatment of the baby are in question. This is a very scary hypothetical situation, and one that has the potential to occur. For these reasons, we feel it is important to become versed in the legal language necessary to protect your rights.

In the above scenario, it would be important to have legal documents in place that specify each partner's right to make decisions in life-threatening situations, when either partner is deemed incompetent or unable to make or articulate decisions for herself. A living will, power of attorney, and last will and testament are three documents that seem essential in this day and age. Because lesbian partners' rights are not automatic, like heterosexual married couples' are, we must take extra care to plan for the unexpected so that our individual wishes are protected and so that our partners can make decisions on our behalf.

With regard to securing legal parental rights to the baby born from DI, there are several options to consider. The biological mother, the mother who physically carries and delivers the baby, is considered legally, upon birth, the only parent of the baby. The nonbiological parent, while a parent in every sense of the word in lesbian couples' minds, must take legal steps to cement her tie to the child in a court of law. She may have the option of pursuing a legal guardianship (depending on the state of residence), which basically grants her the legal right to act as the child's parent at any time (making medical decisions, talking with teachers at school, authorizing permissions for miscellaneous things, perhaps carrying the child on her health insurance through work, etc.). The one limitation, which is an important one, is that a legal guardian's rights can be contested if the biological mother dies. Thus, a legal guardianship is not a *permanent* parental right. It grants more legal equality and protection when compared to having nothing in place at all, but it still has its limitations. Another option that may find legal recognition in your state is processing a parenting agreement with an attorney. This agreement often ties parents together in a joint pledge to be financially responsible for the child; therefore, it may be considered legally binding.

The third option is adoption. Different states vary as to what they call this proceeding and how it is processed. Some states require that for an adoption petition, the parental rights of the biological mother have to be terminated before a joint adoption for both parents is granted. We have heard attorneys discuss this option, and it is our understanding that the biological mother's rights are terminated for literally a few minutes, leaving the baby a ward of the state for that brief moment in time. Then paperwork is signed granting both parents the adoption. Thus, both parents are then adoptive parents with the same rights as any other adoptive or biological couple.

A fourth and, as we see it, most ideal option is to petition for a co-adoption. With a co-adoption, or joint adoption, the biological parent maintains her parental rights to the child, so no rights are ever terminated. And the nonbiological parent merely acquires joint rights to the child, as if the baby were her own, biologically. If a co-adoption is granted, it is a permanent decision and right.

In order to process petitions for a legal guardianship or parenting agreement, your attorneys generally can draw up the paperwork, file it with the court, and often avoid any formal hearing. Guardianships and parenting agreements are either granted or denied.

In order to process an adoption, the following steps might be taken (not necessarily in this order):

- Your attorneys will draw up the appropriate paperwork.
- The nonbiological parent will need to have a certain number of people provide character reference letters on her behalf (generally six people, 2-3 who have known her for more than five years).
- The nonbiological parent will need to have a wellness physical conducted by her physician, basically stating that she is in good physical health.
- Both the nonbiological parent and the biological parent might need to provide criminal background clearances and child sexual abuse clearances from the state.
- Often, a home study performed by a licensed mental health professional is required.

- The attorneys collect and organize all of the appropriate documentation and submit it to the court. They await a date to present the petition to a judge, who will determine whether he/she will even hear the
case and consider the adoption.
- If the judge denies the petition for a hearing, you can either appeal
the decision or accept the judgment.
- If the judge grants the petition for an adoption hearing, a date will be
set for the hearing, which all parties will have to attend. The biological
parent, the nonbiological parent, supportive character witnesses,
etc., will all likely be required to testify at the adoption hearing.
- The necessary parties will testify, and the judge will then make a ruling.
- This ruling can be accepted by the parents or appealed.

These options are presented for you to consider, and, if you are interested,
to consult with an attorney to clarify and verify the specifics about proceed-
ings in your local court system and within your state. The fees for these services vary from attorney to attorney, and that is something else that we
recommend you investigate.

Given the uncertainty of the law, the rights of lesbian couples, and homosexual adoptions in this country, one other option to consider might be to file
for a legal guardianship (which sometimes is easier to obtain than a
co-adoption), or its equivalent in your state, to secure protection for the
nonbiological parent and her rights to the child at least in some capacity.
Then, once that is secured, proceed if you desire with the petition for adoption. This may reduce the emotional tension surrounding the bigger question of whether or not an adoption will be granted by solidifying a legal
connection between the nonbiological partner and the baby/child.

Just as has been required of you and your partner throughout the DI
process, the legal aspects of parenting require a great deal of self-education
and scrutiny. Whether or not you pursue a guardianship or adoption, in
our hearts, lesbian women and their children will always be a family. But it
sure is an incredible feeling to have the law on your side.

Chapter Fourteen

A Conception Recipe

While it is clear that donor insemination is not for the weak-hearted, it is a viable path to parenthood for lesbian women. In the end, only one of millions and millions of sperm has to reach the egg and form a union to create the little person whom we have waited our entire lives to meet. And that, our friends, is certainly worth waiting for.

In this final chapter, we have prepared a *conception recipe*: a fertility and conception checklist. While the information provided in each of the previous chapters is much more thorough, we will provide a brief summary of the essential components of the process as well as a quick reference checklist to help you organize your insemination plans.

We will begin with the signs of fertility. Before beginning the inseminations, you will need to track your ovulation in order to identify your basic menstrual patterns over time. To do this, you must assemble your fertility "kit." In your kit, you will need: a basal temperature chart, pen, a thermometer (a high-quality name-brand digital thermometer or a mercury-based, basal thermometer), and an ovulation predictor kit. You will monitor your BBT, the quantity and quality of your CM, and the positioning and opening of the Os, recording daily findings on the chart. You will complement this record using your ovulation predictor kit (per the manufacturer's instructions). Ideally, three cycles will be tracked in order to establish these patterns.

To those women who intend to consider and take a fertility medication, discuss your options with your doctor. If one is prescribed, follow your doctor's instructions as to how and when you take the medication.

It is during this three-cycle fertility assessment that you will gather information en route to choosing a donor. Based on the fertility data you are collecting, and your own personal preferences, you will choose a known or unknown donor, how many samples/vials per month you will inseminate, and your optimal days of insemination. If you are working with a known donor, you will draw up a sperm sale agreement, a known donor agreement, and, if applicable, a parenting agreement. If you are working with an unknown donor, you will choose a physician, cryobank, and donor. For work with either donor type, you will select your method of insemination: IVI, ICI, or IUI. Shipping/delivery arrangements will be made. If applicable, your doctors will be placed on alert to expect your call requesting an appointment within your ovulation window.

Once your fertility pattern is identified and your donor and insemination method are selected, you then will actually plan your inseminations. You will begin testing with the ovulation predictor kit as instructed. When the LH surge is identified via a positive test result, you either contact your known donor and arrange for semen deliveries, or you arrange the shipment of your cryobank's samples while contacting your doctor and making an appointment for in-office inseminations the following two mornings. After each insemination, you will lie flat on your back with your hips elevated, if possible for a minimum of twenty to thirty minutes (and otherwise, for as long as possible). Document insemination dates on your chart.

Once inseminations are performed during your peak ovulation window, you will continue tracking your BBT, CM, and Os through the anticipated dates of your period. If your temperature dips down at the end of the cycle, prepare for the possibility of your period and planning the next month's cycle. If your temperature remains high well beyond the dates of your expected period, break out your at-home pregnancy test and follow the instructions and/or call your doctor. If it is positive, it is time to celebrate!

If all conditions are optimal, there is a good chance of conception. Silber (1980) describes this as a "game of odds," which may help you to understand your chances of conception (p. 56). Each of these ingredients is important to the conception recipe. And with each insemination, there is a chance of conception. When mixed together in a homeostatic environment, these essential ingredients can combine to form the most precious little being ever to enter your life. And this is what donor insemination is all about.

Lesbian women *are* having babies. We are enduring societal pressures, fertility questions, financial constraints, and emotional and physical stress because of our deep commitment to family. And it's working. The reason for this, we can only assume, is that lesbian women are working with some wonderful known donors and/or establishing relationships with the physicians who are facilitating their families, all the while educating themselves on the critical timing of DI. We are learning to maximize the 48-72 hour peak fertility window and not to waste a precious drop of the essential semen. We are smart, capable, and in control of our own fertility.

This is an exciting time. We hope that the material presented in this book has helped to clarify some of your donor insemination questions and that you can learn from our "trial and error" methods, our failures, and our successes. As we adoringly love our two sons, we join all lesbian women in the quest to create family in our own way, on our own terms. Best of luck in this process, and congratulations to lesbian moms everywhere on the birth of your families!

A CONCEPTION RECIPE

A Quick Reference List

Have?	**Fertility Tracking**
Y or N	Basal temperature chart and pen
Y or N	Thermometer (digital or mercury-based)
Y or N	Daily record of quantity and quality of cervical mucus
Y or N	Daily check of the cervical opening, or Os
Y or N	5-day ovulation predictor test kit

Fertility Medication

Y or N	Consult arranged with doctor about fertility drugs
Y or N	Decision made about whether or not to take medication
Y or N	Have understanding about how and when to take medication, if applicable

Sperm Selection Recipe

Y or N	Path chosen: ___Unknown donor ___Known donor
Y or N	Rank-ordered desirable donor characteristics

_____Clean medical history	_____Ethnic origin
_____Height-weight ratio	_____Eye and hair color
_____Personality	_____Intelligence (grade
	pt. avg./high test scores)
_____Hobbies	_____Other_____

Y or N	*Unknown donor* selected
	If yes, name physician, cryobank, donor #, and insemination type:
	_____
Y or N	*Known donor* selected
	If yes, name donor, physician (if applicable), and insemination type:
	_____
Y or N	Monthly budget constructed, for sperm and insemination expenses
Y or N	Sperm sample delivery arrangements made:
	Unknown donor–Cryobank shipping procedures and fees are understood and arranged, if applicable
	Known donor–Arrangements have been made with donor as to the appropriate ways to obtain and store sample for delivery during fertile "window"

Have?	Ultimate Conception Recipe
Y or N	Insemination consultation secured with primary care physician or ob-gyn/fertility doctor
Y or N	Mutual love, affection, and support offered and experienced by both partners
Y or N	Decision made to pursue DI, together
Y or N	Efforts to maintain *womb wellness* pursued and achieved
Y or N	Daily prenatal vitamin taken (preferably 3 months prior to inseminations)
Y or N	BBT, CM, Os, and OPK results recorded on temperature chart
Y or N	If applicable, cryobank selected and account established
Y or N	If applicable, physician selected and insemination plan discussed
Y or N	Donor selected–appropriate fees paid and agreements made
Y or N	Positive ovulation predictor test secured
Y or N	2 IUI inseminations conducted, 24 hours apart (frozen semen) or 2 IVI or IUI inseminations, 36-48 hours apart (fresh semen)
Y or N	Continued BBT, CM, and Os tracking
Y or N	Temperature graph on chart dropped at end of cycle–period imminent
Y or N	Temperature remained high–pregnancy imminent! (If yes, make appointment with doctor for blood test to confirm)

GOOD LUCK!

Bibliography

Clunis, D. Merilee & Green, G. Dorsey. (1995). *The lesbian parenting book: A guide to creating families and raising children*. Seattle, WA: Seal Press.

Curry, Hayden, Clifford, Denis, & Leonard, Robin. (1994). *A legal guide for lesbian and gay couples*. Berkeley, CA: Nolo Press.

Eisenberg, Arlene, Murkoff, Heidi E., & Hathaway, Sandee E., B.S.N. (1991). *What to expect when you're expecting*. New York, NY: Workman Publishing Company, Inc.

Lauersen, Niels H., M.D., Ph.D., & Bouchez, Colette. (1991). *Getting pregnant: What couples need to know right now*. New York: Ballantine Books.

Mohler, Marie, M.A. (1999). *Homosexual rites of passage: A road to visibility and validation*. Binghamton, NY: Harrington Park Press.

Noble, Elizabeth. (1987). *Having your baby by donor insemination: A complete resource guide*. Boston, MA: Houghton Mifflin Company.

Nofziger, Margaret. (1982). *The fertility question*. Summertown, TN: The Book Publishing Co.

Nofziger, Margaret. (1992). *A cooperative method of natural birth control*. Summertown, TN: The Book Publishing Co.

Nofziger, Margaret. (1998). *Signs of fertility: The personal science of natural birth control*. Deatsville, AL: MND Publishing, Inc.

Silber, Sherman J., M.D. (1980). *How to get pregnant*. New York, NY: Warner Books, Inc.

Sperm Bank of California. (Winter 1999). Newsletter article: *Fertility awareness is step one*. Vol. V, No. 1.

Sussman, John R., M.D., & Levitt, B. Blake. (1989). *Before you conceive: The complete prepregnancy guide*. New York, NY: Bantam Books.

The California Cryobank marketing materials. (1998).

The Fairfax Cryobank marketing materials. (1999).

APPENDICES

APPENDIX A

Sample Basal Temperature Chart

Month:																																									
Date																																										
Day of Cycle	1	2	3	4	5	6	7	8	9	10	11	12	13	14	15	16	17	18	19	20	21	22	23	24	25	26	27	28	29	30	31	32	33	34	35	36	37	38	39	40	41	42
Insemination																																										
Menses																																										
Medication																																										

Temperature scale (rows): 99.0, .9, .8, .7, .6, .5, .4, .3, .2, .1, 98.0, .9, .8, .7, .6, .5, .4, .3, .2, .1, 97.0

CM & Os Notes

APPENDIX B

Ovulatory Cycle–No Pregnancy (Ovulation Around Cycle Days 15-16)

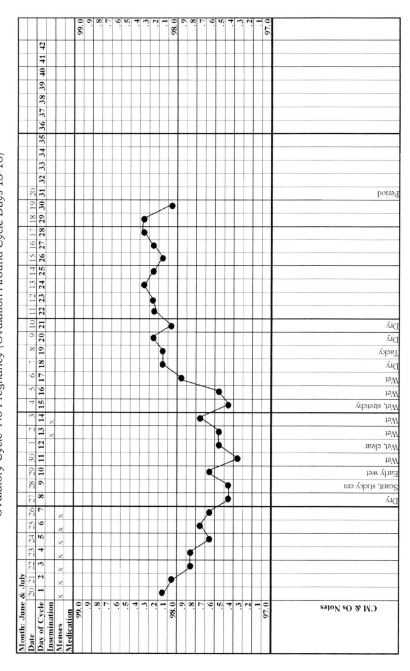

APPENDIX C
Anovulatory Cycle (No Ovulation, No Pregnancy)

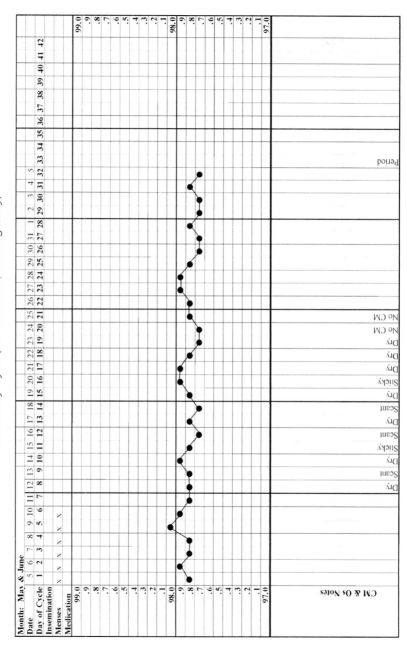

APPENDIX D

Ovulatory Cycle–Pregnancy Achieved (Ovulation Around Cycle Days 13 and 14)

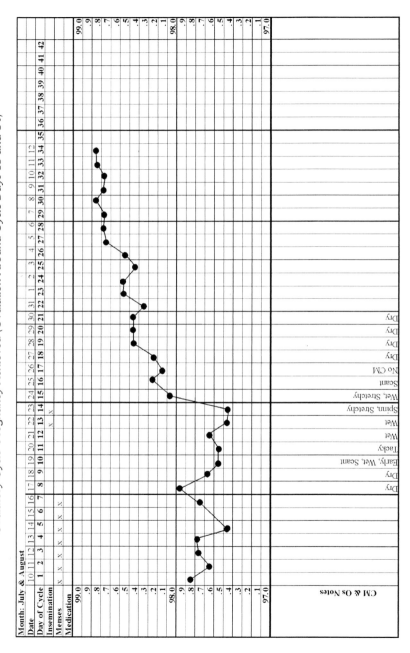

About the Authors

Marie Mohler, MA, is a professional counselor and author. After completing her master's degree in psychology in 1997, she worked for several years as a family therapist for a large, non-profit organization in the Pittsburgh, Pennsylvania, area. Her first book was *Homosexual Rites of Passage: A Road to Visibility and Validation* (Harrington Park Press, 1999). Ms. Mohler's commitment to the lesbian community is evident in her latest work in progress, a newsletter tentatively entitled *The Lavender Lighthouse: Helping Women Navigate Donor Insemination, Pregnancy, and Parenthood.* This literary forum is intended to serve as an extension of this book by inviting lesbian women and parents to share their wisdom, fears, challenges, and successes with one another. For more information on her newsletter, please send an e-mail to <lavenderlighthouse@yahoo. com>. Those interested in a personalized DI consult and/or ongoing support can send an e-mail to Ms. Mohler at <dicoaching@yahoo. com>.

Lacy Frazer, PsyD, earned her doctorate in clinical psychology from the Georgia School of Professional Psychology in 1997. She currently works as a clinical psychologist in a correctional setting. Dr. Frazer and Ms. Mohler share a life partnership of ten years and co-parent two sons conceived through donor insemination. Their family lives in Durham, North Carolina.